D1320943

A Year in the Life of the Animal Hospital

David Grant

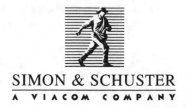

SIMON & SCHUSTER
A VIACOM COMPANY

First published in Great Britain
by Simon & Schuster UK Ltd, 1998

A Viacom company

Copyright © David Grant, 1998

This book is copyright under the Berne Convention.
No reproduction without permission.

All rights reserved

The right of David Grant to be identified as author of this work
has been asserted by him in accordance with sections 77 and 78
of the Copyright, Designs and Patents Act, 1988

1 3 5 7 9 10 8 6 4 2

Simon & Schuster UK Ltd
Africa House
64-78 Kingsway
London WC2B 6AH

Simon & Schuster Australia
Sydney

A CIP catalogue record for this book is available from the British Library

ISBN 0-684-85141-5

Typeset by SX Composing DTP., Rayleigh, Essex
Printed and bound in Great Britain by
Butler & Tanner Ltd., Frome, Somerset

To Rachel, Laura and Ellie

Also by David Grant

Tales from the Animal Hospital

ACKNOWLEDGEMENTS

Thanks to Helen Gummer, Ingrid Connell and Aruna Mathur and all the staff at Simon & Schuster

AUTHOR'S NOTE

Although all the stories that feature in this book are true, the names of pets and owners have been changed to protect their privacy.

CONTENTS

JANUARY

January 1 is never a particularly arduous day to be on duty. Most people don't seem to surface until the afternoon, and the day tends to be quiet. As on all bank holidays (and weekends, too) we can manage with emergency-only surgeries with only one veterinary surgeon on duty. This was me, and as I started a new year in the animal hospital I didn't expect the day to be too busy – based on past experience. Little did I know!

Having had a week off over Christmas, I arrived at the hospital to find that the winter had already taken its toll on our nurses. Half a dozen were off sick with a nasty flu bug and it was a skeleton crew that were going to get through the day's emergencies with me: just three nurses for the morning and afternoon session, three until late evening and two overnight. This would put them under pressure if we had a rush of cases during the day.

If we were hoping for a quiet time the omens were not good because, within five minutes of my arrival, the first emergency was on the scene: a small black and white cat, only eight months old – too young to be pregnant – was trying unsuccessfully to give birth. She had been at it all night and it was obvious to her owners, Colin and Julie, that things weren't progressing normally. By coincidence their baby had only just come out of the special-care unit and I knew about all the stress that that entails. My first daughter had entered the world prematurely on a New Year's Eve

1

and my first real sight of her had been a shock. She was in intensive care, surrounded by a baffling array of high-tech equipment. A machine was breathing for her through a tube into her lungs, which were too immature to function by themselves. To prevent her pulling out the tubes another machine gave minute doses of morphine at intervals into her vein. This made her very dopey. We were told by the staff to talk to her lots even though she was just born, as babies of this age do respond to voices. I shall never forget the way her eyes struggled to open as I called her name. It was a long week of sleepless nights and a lesson in caring from those wonderful special-care doctors and nurses.

I understood what Colin and Julie had been through and I wasn't surprised that they hadn't got round to having Bonny spayed, which would normally be done at five months. She must have got pregnant before she was even six months old and now here she was on the examining table straining away with an anxious look on her face. She would need an immediate Caesarean and Colin and Julie signed the consent form then sat down in Reception to wait.

Half an hour later I had brought four weak-looking kittens into the world. Bonny was still blissfully asleep so I put the kittens separately in another cage with a hot-water bottle. As I looked down on them I wondered if they would survive. No high-tech equipment, no tubes into their lungs, just the warmth and care of their mother – assuming that she would take to them.

Over the years I have seen many instances of an apparent refusal by the mother to have anything to do with her litter. On the other hand, I have also seen the total devotion of a friend's cat, Mini, to her newborn. Mini had been hand-reared since birth when her mother abandoned her. A couple of the nurses took her on and spent days and nights feeding her. She was quite poorly for a month then finally turned the corner, although she never really caught up as far as size was concerned: at a year old she looked about six months – hence her name. At last my friend thought she was putting on weight and getting bigger but in reality Mini was pregnant. This was a real surprise since she had never shown any sign of being in season. When it became obvious that she wasn't going to grow any more she had been scheduled for spaying. When she had her litter they were soon nearly as big as her. In spite of never having benefited from a natural mother herself, she was magnificent at parenthood and three kittens grew up into fine, healthy, well-adapted specimens – although, curiously, she refused to feed a fourth.

If my New Year kittens were to survive they would need to be put in with their mother as soon as possible. The outlook didn't look good because although they were breathing on their own they weren't crying or trying to move about. As soon as Bonny came round from the anaesthetic they were put with her. A couple of the nurses and I watched anxiously as she sniffed at the kittens then began to lick and nuzzle them. So far so good! And if they survived we knew good homes were being organised for them by Colin and Julie. I told the young couple to go home now and promised we would let them know by the end of the day how Bonny and her kittens were getting on.

The newborn kittens weren't the only ones to end up in the hospital that day: there was a grand total of twenty-five – most of them abandoned. The usual post-Christmas rush. Well, they could wait in the hospital until we could phone round the homing centres next week and I was fairly confident that we would place them somewhere. One particularly cute ginger tom caught my eye. He was scaling his cage like

3

a rock-climber while the nurses took turns to tickle his tummy. I was tempted to take him home – a feeling that hits me every week. And it wasn't just the kitten who caught my eye. We had an influx of dogs too – six stray puppies and a couple of old German shepherd dogs, both obviously owned but with no identification. They would be collected by the Battersea Dogs' Home tomorrow. Goodness knows why the poor dogs had been abandoned since they were both of a delightful temperament.

All in all it was not a good start to the year and it was still only ten in the morning. I could tell, from their unusually subdued moods, that one or two of the nurses were feeling sad. Later on they cheered up when I reminded them that we usually managed to get strays into homing centres with great success at this time of year. It's very hard on the nurses having to care for so many poor animals who have never known true human kindness, to see them respond and then, at the end of the day, not to know the outcome – whether the cat or dog they had fallen in love with would find a good home.

I had managed to get the owned animals in the hospital home for Christmas so apart from the strays there weren't many animals in, but another pet was waiting in the emergency surgery. This was Bob, a young collie cross, who had never been to us before. Helen, his owner, was a bit embarrassed about coming to the emergency service as his problem had started a few days earlier, but it was soon apparent that it needed sorting out right away.

Three or four days before Bob had pinched the remains of the family Christmas turkey and demolished the lot – bones and all. Within a day he was straining to pass motions and liberal doses of liquid paraffin had failed to help. So here he was on New Year's Day in need of urgent attention.

He stood placidly while I squeezed his tummy gently. Straight away I could feel a hard lump, which was evidently painful. A rectal examination confirmed the worst: lots of minute bone spicules and severe constipation. There was nothing for it: Bob would need an enema. I groaned for his sake and mine.

After giving him an anaesthetic I passed a plastic tube into his bottom and started to pump in liquid paraffin while massaging the lumps. Slowly but surely we cleared the obstruction and cleaned him up. A messy, smelly, unpleasant task. At least the poor dog would feel greatly relieved when he came round. Even though it was cold outside we were glad to work with the windows open – not the best job to have to do before lunch. It was going to be one of those days.

No sooner was Bob starting to come round in Ward One than Jenny, the duty nurse on Reception, phoned through to the theatre to say that a 'fitting' dog was coming in. It's a common problem and we have lots of epileptic dogs on the files who have to have regular medication. From what Jenny had been able to find out from the distressed owners, it was a German shepherd of about two years old. It had been having continuous fits since first thing that morning. Jenny calmed the owners, got them to wrap the dog warmly in a large blanket and start out for the hospital.

There is a standard way of dealing with such cases, which makes things relatively easy, but while waiting for the dog's arrival my mind went back to my first such case, twenty-five years before, when I did my first stint at the Harmsworth Hospital as a young recently qualified vet. It was another German shepherd, which had been fitting on and off all day. This is a condition called *status epilepticus* and is a real emergency as death can result unless the fits are stopped. Kaiser had been on treatment for some time but that day had suddenly deteriorated. He came in only semi-conscious, shaking and drooling. Every few minutes he would go into a full-blown fit, which would last about two minutes. In the end I had to resort to deep anaesthesia with pentobarbitone into the vein. Pentobarbitone was the first intravenous anaesthetic to be developed but it is so long-acting that it is not used now for routine anaesthesia. Kaiser would be under for eight hours or so but every time he started to come round his fits began again. All in all he was kept anaesthetised for more than forty-eight hours but it took a week before we managed to stabilize him on new medication. I remember him now, a beautiful, placid animal. To say that his owner, John, was over the moon was a real understatement.

I stayed another three years at the Harmsworth and I saw Kaiser regularly. He didn't have a repetition of his *status epilepticus* and went on to live another ten years with his epilepsy well controlled. We didn't know a lot about the disease in young dogs then and still don't now. Cases like Kaiser's are referred to as 'idiopathic' epilepsy, which is a fancy way of saying we don't know the cause. For years afterwards John sent chocolates to the nurses at Christmas for he recognized that they had played a major part in his dog's recovery.

A screech of brakes heralded the arrival of our 'fitting' patient. His owners, the Browns, a couple with three children, were relieved to see Jenny and Liz who had gone straight out with the trolley to help get the dog admitted, not an easy task since he was trembling and convulsing inter-mittently. He was wheeled straight down to the prep room, where I was waiting with a couple of vials of Valium. Nowadays this is the first choice to stop the fits and, with a bit of a struggle and with the nurses holding him down as best they could, I managed to get some slowly into the dog's vein. The effect was immediate and gratifying. As he went under he gave a sigh and relaxed, taking deep, regular breaths. Keeping the needle in the vein I took some blood to check his liver function, since liver disease can sometimes be a cause of fits. Meanwhile, Jenny and Liz, with their usual efficiency, had set up a drip to keep the dog's fluid balance correct over the next day or so. Having a line into the vein would also mean that it would be easy to give him more Valium later if he needed it. Quite often, in cases like this, it takes two or three days, or even longer, to get things under control – just as with Kaiser all those years ago.

With the panic over, I had time to write up the notes and prepare reports – and saw the second coincidence of the day! That dog's name was Kaiser and he was two years old. Still, but lots of German shepherd dogs are called Kaiser, and two years is a common age for epilepsy to start in this breed.

By now it was getting on for two o'clock and I headed home for lunch – just a twelve-minute journey with the roads so quiet. With a mobile phone – one luxury we didn't have twenty-five years ago – we have the freedom to move about yet be immediately available for advice. It was bliss to have something to eat and put my feet up for an hour or so – I have learned that it's best to pace yourself on duty and take rest when you can. It's so easy to become exhausted when on twenty-four-hour duty if you don't try to set aside rest periods.

Meanwhile, back at the hospital, the shift nurses, or 'shifties' as they get called, would be busy assessing the by now constant stream of 'emergencies' coming through the door. They would call me for anything urgent and I could be there quickly, but most cases could wait and we would see them in a mini-session later on. A good 90 per cent of cases during emergency hours aren't true emergencies, as I demonstrated later in the clinic.

At five p.m. I was back, assessing the afternoon's list. As usual this was about ten cases long but none were life-threatening, although some were more urgent than others. One of the more unusual cases was Buster, a normally bouncing mongrel full of life, who had been adopted from the Battersea Dogs' Home. I put him at about eighteen months old, based on his strong healthy teeth. Just the age for getting up to all sorts of mischief. I had seen him several times before, usually with tummy upsets. His zest for life included a great love of food – especially chocolate. This he shared with me! Unlike me, however (although some would say otherwise), Buster didn't know when to stop. Just like Bob he was a victim of post-Christmas gluttony – in his case a large box of dark chocolates.

He had eaten them in the morning and at first the owners had thought nothing of it, but later Buster started to look a bit jittery and had a bad attack of diarrhoea. When I examined him he was looking even more sorry for himself, with tummy pain and loss of bladder control. It looked as though the chocolates were to blame. I hurried away to my book on poisoning to see what, if anything, it said about chocolate poisoning – I hadn't encountered it before. You can imagine my surprise when I read that it was most common in dogs. The active ingredient that causes the illness is theobromine, which belongs to a class of drugs commonly used to treat heart disease. I looked up the symptoms: thirst, tummy upsets, loss of bladder control, agitation and nervousness, a racing heart – and, in extreme cases, coma and death. The book even had the approximate dose to cause symptoms: 1.3mg/kg of baker's chocolate. I was intrigued to read that the risk of poisoning from milk chocolate was about ten times less as it contains much less theobromine.

On taking another look at Buster, I found his heart was racing away at 140 beats per minute. Everything fitted. I thought it was too late to make him sick so I elected to put him on a drip to counter any fluid imbalance from the diarrhoea and loss of bladder control, and gave him some mild sedative to counteract his jittery anxious behaviour. He was admitted for observation.

Next came a couple of stitch-ups: a cat had caught herself on something – a nail in all probability – and a dog had been badly bitten. Twenty stitches later, the latter was waking up and I was ready for the evening session. These patients had been selected in order of urgency by the experienced nurses, a process called triage. It wasn't a term with which I was familiar until I had to go several times to the casualty clinic with one or other of my daughters. I was amazed by what I saw: crowds of people with no discernible life-threatening illness. In fact, I heard one young lad, who had turned up with his girlfriend, complaining that his sore throat of two days' duration was getting worse and asking if he could be seen immediately.

One of the less urgent cases was a Labrador called Sooty, who had been limping off and on for six weeks. His owners, an elderly couple called Dot and Bert, had struggled in, walking the three miles to the hospital as they lacked their own transport. As they sat in the waiting room, flushed and tired, I hadn't the heart to ask why they hadn't come earlier. And the best of it was that when I examined Sooty I couldn't find anything wrong – in fact, he wasn't even lame. Dot explained that his lameness usually got better with exercise! Sooty was twelve and I thought that he probably had mild arthritis – not uncommon in older dogs

9

(or senior dogs as the Americans call them). He flinched when I felt round his hips, which confirmed my diagnosis. I started him on some arthritis pills and suggested his owners try to get hold of a friend to give them a lift home. 'Could you come to normal surgery next time?' I asked politely – no point being miffed on the first day of the year!

Half an hour later I had sorted out a collection of tummy upsets, earaches and skin infections and was ready to set off for home where I would spend the rest of the night, hopefully, on standby. First I looked at Bonny, our Caesarean of the morning. The kittens were feeding on their purring mother – they would undoubtedly survive! Nature had worked another little miracle and I headed home feeling happy with the day. Even better, there were no phone calls that night and I slept soundly until the alarm woke me at seven the next morning.

My day always starts in more or less the same way. I try to get in early, sometime after eight. It gives me an opportunity to talk without interruption to Sonia, the hospital manager. She has worked at the Harmsworth for more than twenty years and we can talk about virtually anything, from management problems in the hospital to whom to employ as a nurse. She lives some distance away and likes to travel early so she's usually in at around seven or even earlier. First thing in the morning is often the only time we get to talk as we are both so busy. She has to deal with the non-veterinary side of the hospital, which is quite a job. After talking to her, and if the mail is on time, I like to go through the letters and earmark any that require urgent replies.

At around nine I set off on the ward rounds. Wards one and two are for dogs, wards three and four for cats, five and six are isolation cases, seven is mainly used for stray cats, and eight is our 'exotic' ward, which usually contains birds, rabbits, guinea-pigs, hamsters and other small animals. It takes about an hour to check on all the patients and discharge those which can go home – getting them off the premises as soon as they are well enough is crucial as we need the 'beds' for in-coming patients. It's just like the NHS in miniature. It can be difficult when we are very busy in the summer, even though, when pushed, we can hospitalize 110 animals.

On the ward rounds I was delighted to see that Buster, the chocoholic, had made an almost miraculous recovery. His heart-rate was back to normal and he was bright-eyed and exuberant, barking furiously for breakfast. I thought it safe enough to ask the nurses to prepare him some chicken, which disappeared in about ten seconds. He could go home that afternoon if there were no further problems.

By now my colleagues had arrived. Jeremy was busy consulting. The numbers are always up after a bank holiday and forty patients were waiting for him. There would be no chance to wish him a happy new year until the afternoon. Bairbre was out at our clinic in Kilburn and lucky old Stan was still at home in Barbados. He wouldn't be back at work for a couple of days. That left Helen, Gabriel and me to get through the morning's operating list. The day was so busy we caught only fleeting glimpses of each other, with barely time to ask how the holidays had gone. How quickly life gets back to normal after Christmas.

That week flu continued to take its toll of the nurses, and as one came back to work another would go down with it. Several operations had to be cancelled. Then several stray cats went down with the feline version of flu. This is always a nuisance since it means that we can't get them into homing centres until they recover, which they usually do.

11

Cat flu is not a true influenza virus but the signs are similar to the human disease.

In ward seven I checked over a black and white kitten, which had just gone down with the typical symptoms. She was sneezing, had a sore, runny eye and a red, angry-looking ulcer on her tongue. Poor little thing. She had been in the hospital only a few days so had obviously been incubating it from her previous home. She had no identification and it was highly unlikely that anyone had ever bothered to have her vaccinated. The treatment for these cases is straightforward: antibiotics to prevent secondary infection, eye ointment and good nursing. She was transferred to the isolation ward and I kept my fingers crossed for her. We can sometimes cure and rehome animals that have been in isolation but it is quite difficult, mainly because they sometimes have residual occasional sneezing, which means that we can't be sure that they are no longer infectious. Cat flu is rarely fatal and, with treatment, will normally get better within ten days or so, but that is much more likely in a proper caring home. Even though the nurses do a wonderful job, it is much harder to cure cat flu in hospital. I have never been sure why this is: perhaps, in spite of the wonderful attention they get, the stress of being in hospital works against the healing process. My wife's cat, Penny, had been rescued from here and made a full recovery, but only after we took her home where she had personal undivided attention and nursing plus lots of fresh air.

Before I had finished the ward rounds the black and white kitten's fortunes had been transformed: one of the RSPCA's branch workers had spotted her and taken her on. Gloria was always helping us like this and I couldn't thank her enough.

The second week brought winter and its own problems.

It had been unseasonably mild and, as an avid weather-watcher, I had been waiting for the sudden change. With my television on the blink – my youngest had posted a large number of objects into the video – I hadn't been doing my usual three-times-daily weather-forecast viewing and on Monday morning I was surprised to wake up to heavy snow. The roads around my home were just about all right but many of our staff live quite far away and had trouble travelling in. Thankfully, the same was true of the owners, whose numbers were reduced to a trickle. Only the locals ventured out.

Snow and ice bring all sorts of problems to humans and animals. Early that morning one man had taken his dog, Lassie, out and she had become very lame on one of her front paws. I soon found the cause of the problem: it was a large ice ball, embedded between her pads. This would have sorted itself out if she had just stayed in the warm for twenty minutes – but the poor worried owner struggled to the hospital, walking for half an hour with his dog's problem getting worse by the minute! It was a two-second job to pick out the ice ball. Sometimes the salt put down to keep the snow from settling on the roads can cause dermatitis in the paws, and as a precaution I gave Lassie an anti-inflammatory injection and some antibiotics.

The snow continued to fall, and I was wondering about my journey home when RSPCA Inspector John Bowe rushed into the prep room with three hypothermic kittens. Their plaintive miaows had drawn attention to them: they had been found in a black bag in the rubbish chute of a nearby estate. It's hard to say how long they had been there but they were extremely cold: their temperatures failed to register on the thermometer's scale. In spite of this, they were surprisingly bright and very lucky. I would have given them no chance if they had spent another hour or two in the sub-zero conditions. As it was, they were wrapped quickly in blankets and placed on hot-water bottles. Pretty soon they began to move about, miaowing loudly, and were given some kitten food. Within a few hours they were playing, climbing up the bars of their cage, wrestling with each other and doing all the things that kittens are supposed to do – and causing endless amusement to the nurses who had been able to get in.

I retired to my office to catch up on all the correspondence and paperwork and bask in the luxurious warmth. Thank goodness for efficient central heating. The stray animals at the Harmsworth were definitely in the lap of luxury compared to their unfortunate friends outside.

During the afternoon the snow stopped and more people ventured out, which led to a steady trickle of consultations that the owners felt couldn't wait – although I felt that in the majority of cases it would have been better to nurse the pet at home: the cold outside might have made matters worse. Still, nobody worries more than pet owners – except parents, perhaps!

The cold snap lasted a few days and then, as so often happens, the winds veered round to the south. Suddenly it felt incredibly warm and there was an overnight thaw. We were worked off our feet, day and night, until the end of the week. One dog stands out in my mind, an old Labrador called Sam. He had come in six months earlier with a mild infection in both his ears. This had cleared up quickly with drops but it was obvious that his hearing was on the wane. First, if the television was on, he had stopped responding to the doorbell and later had gone totally deaf. An examination revealed nothing of significance and I just had to put it down to old age. The same thing had happened to my dog

Barney in the last year of his life – I had had to draw his attention by touching him or waving at him. He really turned into an old gentleman in many ways.

Sam lived alone with his owner, Geoff, who was in his eighties. Geoff was not at all worried by the poor outlook I had given as far as Sam's hearing was concerned. 'I'll teach him sign language,' he told me confidently. And here Sam was, six months later, having a check-up for a cough. In a dog of Sam's age – fourteen – the heart was the first thing to look at. Sure enough, instead of the steady sharp clicking of normal heart valves opening and snapping shut, I could hear the characteristic whoosh-whoosh sound caused by damaged valves with blood leaking through them at each beat. The net result is an inefficient heart that does not produce enough pressure, and one of the first signs is a build-up of fluid in the lungs, which causes a cough. Sam was absolutely typical: his cough was worse at night when he was lying down, which contributes to the collection of fluid in his lungs, and also when he tried to run or got excited. The diagnosis can be confirmed by taking an X-ray of the chest, which will show the heart's attempt to compensate by enlarging to try to pump more blood into the circulation. In Sam's case this could be done without an anaesthetic.

Since I had last seen him, Geoff had indeed succeeded in teaching Sam sign language. He had already demonstrated it to me: as they arrived, Geoff pointed down and Sam immediately sat. He did it again on the consulting table – quite an achievement since most dogs panic in this most stressful situation! When I wanted Sam to lie down I moved my hand palm down and he did as asked. All in all Sam had learned to sit, stay, come, roll over and give his paw by sign language. In a space of six months. Almost to show off, Geoff gave a circular motion of his hand and

Sam lay on his side. This made examination of the left part of the heart, the usual seat of the problem, quite easy. Sam even obeyed these signs when Geoff wasn't giving them. Half an hour later I was tickled pink when, at my gesture, he rolled over on to his side on the X-ray table. A press of the button from behind the lead screen and the X-ray had been taken.

A few minutes later, as I looked at the X-ray plate, the diagnosis of leaky heart valves leading to congestive heart failure was confirmed. The response to treatment for this is almost always excellent, though, as I explained to Geoff. Sam would be given a drug called frusemide, which helps to remove fluid from the lungs, and another called amino-phylline, a heart stimulant – in the same class as the drug found in chocolate that had caused Buster's problem. I fully expected the cough to go and Sam's exercise tolerance to improve.

Later I found out that my confidence had been justified. One day a box of biscuits appeared and I was told that Geoff had brought them in as a thank-you for the nurses. On checking his file, I noted that Stan had seen Sam for a check-up and everything was going well. I was pleased for Geoff and Sam – and having seen the astonishing way that Sam had learned sign language, I had to revise my opinion that it was difficult to teach an old dog new tricks!

The next day on ward rounds the reports nurse was Clare, who is always cheerful and chatty. This particular Tuesday she was on top form, and when I asked her why she told me that the three hypothermic kittens had gone together to a lovely home. Clare's expertise, along with several other nurses, is getting cats out to all the homing centres that the RSPCA runs within striking distance and maintaining good links with her colleagues there. When she hears that things have worked out for a cat or kittens who have plucked at everyone's heartstrings it makes all her considerable efforts worthwhile.

Later that day I became the next victim of flu. Quite suddenly, I had a fever and generalized aches and pains. My temperature shot up and for the first time in years I had to take time off. Vets are generally a hardy lot but I felt so rough I just could not work and that was that.

I had forgotten what it's like to have genuine flu. The last time had probably been when I was at school. I remembered suffering for at least a week and the numbers at school were decimated. Having a constant fever is so unpleasant and any virus leaves me with an intractable cough. I tend to take good health for granted but being ill gave me an insight into my patients. On my return I really sympathized with the assorted dogs, cats and small creatures that formed my first clinic. However, animals seem so much better than humans at resisting illness and they don't dwell on the unpleasantness to such a degree. One thing that never ceases to amaze me is that most human conditions have their parallel in animals, although from my own experience, since having children, more viruses afflict people than animals. Having been illness-free for so many years, I have now lost count of the number of bugs I have caught from my children.

One case that illustrates this point came in towards the end of the month, when I was presented with an interesting eye condition in a cat. Eye conditions are rather complicated and some cases need specialist treatment, especially if surgery is involved. Removing cataracts is routine in human surgery, with good results, but more difficult in dogs and cats, and is usually done by vets with specialist qualifications. A seven-year-old moggy called Little Toby didn't have cataracts, he had something much more painful and something I could relate to myself: about fifteen years before I had suffered from exactly the same condition. Little Toby was in great pain and off his food. Both eyes were screwed up and he couldn't bear the light being shone in them. In fact, he could only just open them. The condition had come on suddenly. He was owned by an elderly couple, Mr and Mrs Smith, who had had cats throughout their married life – all called Little Toby! This one was anything but little: he was a huge, rather fat tabby, the type that loves everyone *and* lots of fuss and stroking. Normally full of life he was utterly dejected as I tried to identify the cause of his pain. With some local anaesthetic drops I was able to get his eyes open. Then I could see that the pupils were tightly constricted and that there was a lot of inflammation in the iris, the coloured part. I put some dye on the outer part of the eye to check for ulceration but there was no sign of this.

It was clear to me that he was suffering from a disease called anterior uveitis, which means inflammation of the front part of the eye. I well remember my experience with this. The pain started inexplicably at about nine in the evening and I took myself to bed with some aspirin. At three the pain was bad enough to wake me up but I soldiered on. By eight the next morning I was just able to get dressed and stagger round to the surgery. The doctor took one look at me and sent me to hospital, offering to call an ambulance, but a colleague's wife drove me there.

Within half an hour of my arrival the senior registrar had made his diagnosis, dilated my pupils with atropine and put in local-anaesthetic drops. Just those two things made the pain much more bearable and, from being virtually unable to walk, I was not far off normal. Suffering severe pain and being relieved of it seems to me to be in some ways a good experience for any doctor or vet since it is bound to put a different perspective on their patients' suffering. Ever since I have been especially sympathetic to pets like Little Toby with the severe pain caused by conditions like anterior uveitis. It is always secondary to a primary disease and to cure the uveitis it is important not only to treat its symptoms but also to investigate the underlying cause. (In my case the underlying cause was never identified in spite of innumerable blood tests.)

Within a week, with atropine drops to keep my pupils dilated, and strong steroids into the eye I was cured and back at work. I prescribed the same treatment for Little Toby and booked him in for a blood test a few days hence. There are many strikingly similar features of the condition in cats and people, the main one being that several diseases are known to underlie it but also that often no cause is found.

I started with a blood test for the leukaemia virus and feline immunodeficiency virus (cat Aids) and a disease called toxoplasmosis, which is common in cats. A few days later, I had the probable answer: Little Toby had proved positive for the Aids virus and negative for everything else. As soon as I reviewed his history with Mr and Mrs Smith the diagnosis made sense. They had rescued Little Toby when he was about two – he had been a stray tom cat, much addicted to fighting. Rescued is perhaps the wrong word: rather, he had adopted the Smiths over a period of time culminating on one vicious winter's day when he had walked into their house, settled down in front of the fire and refused to go out. Then he had been a typically smelly tom cat with an air of neglect about him. Over the next few months, he had been castrated, groomed, and quickly became domesticated, losing his pungent smell. In spite of his reputation – he was known by all the neighbours as a scrapper – he seemed to leave that part of his life behind, preferring the company of his adopted owners and not venturing out much. Latterly he had become a true home lover, only going out in the garden once in a while and never getting into mischief. He had rarely needed the attention of a vet, except for routine vaccinations, and his eye problem was probably the first serious illness he had ever had. It was likely, I told his worried owners, that he had contracted the feline Aids virus in his fighting days since it is mainly transmitted by bite wounds – the virus is found in high concentrations in the saliva. Stray tom cats are particularly at risk from it as they are always fighting.

Feline Aids shares many similarities with the human Aids virus. Fortunately, although they are in the same family they are quite distinct and it is not possible for humans to catch the cat virus. Although first discovered as recently as 1986 the cat Aids virus has been with us much longer than that. Samples of blood taken in 1975 have shown evidence of its presence. When it was discovered, many cat owners were alarmed, understandably, but these days it is not the death sentence to cats that it was once thought to be and many live for years before becoming ill. In many instances I regard it as nothing more than an explanation for certain illnesses – like Little Toby's, for example – or for a cat suffering recurrent illnesses and taking a long time to get over them. At first the Smiths were upset but I reassured them that it was just a question of treating whatever disease cropped up due to the virus weakening the immune system.

A few days later, Little Toby's anterior uveitis was coming nicely under control although, likely as not, he would need constant treatment because we could do nothing to get rid of the Aids virus. In spite of having feline aids it wouldn't surprise me if he went on for some time yet. How long exactly would be very hard to say, though, and I wasn't going to be drawn into any predictions! It's no more easy than winning the lottery. I kept my fingers crossed for him and hoped that he would live for years without further sickness. He would have to be kept indoors to eliminate the risk of him passing the virus on to another cat but that shouldn't be a hardship for such a home-loving cat.

All in all we had been lucky this month. January can be the start of a really hard winter. Cold, exhausted stray cats, unable to survive in the bitter conditions, end up at our door. Wildlife, unable to feed, also arrive in a dangerously weakened state: herons, for example, cannot catch fish if ponds are iced over. This year, the relatively mild weather saw a great reduction in such cases. In fact, the month ended on an optimistic note, with a run of sick pets getting better. Experience had taught me to expect the reverse sooner or later, but for the time being I rejoiced in the knowledge that everything was going well and life seemed almost stress-free. I hoped that February would bring as much fun and satisfaction.

FEBRUARY

February continued mild and we were busy with the usual fascinating variety of cases. A few days into the month I found myself dealing with an interesting rabbit. I have to confess that as a vet I have always found it difficult to get enthusiastic about rabbits as patients. Of course, for many people they are well-loved pets with charming characters, but for me they have a certain impenetrable quality: I can't understand them as I do dogs and cats. You can talk to dogs and cats, fondle them reassuringly and, for the most part, calm them down. I have never been able to do this with rabbits, which must be my fault. They always seem to squirm and jump when I try to examine them and, worse, can sometimes bite without warning. Perhaps the owners should take some of the blame too, though: many rabbits are abandoned to a miserable, lonely existence with little human contact. Small wonder that sometimes they are not easy patients. Increasingly, however, they are kept indoors in a similar way to cats, which has to be more satisfactory for them and, amazingly enough – to me, at any rate – they are apparently not difficult to house-train.

Thumper's contact with humans was *very* intimate, even to the extent of being allowed to sleep in ten-year-old Richard's bed. Many would think that this was going too far, myself included, but if a pet is allowed to get on or in a bed just once, neither child nor animal wants to give it up. Richard was the main reason why Thumper was in the clinic: he had had a troublesome rash for a few weeks, which hadn't responded to treatment, and his doctor suspected that the rabbit might have something to do with it, especially when he found out that Thumper slept in Richard's bed. The rash had spread over much of Richard's tummy and he had been kept away from school, missing a football match as a result, since there was a suspicion that he might have chicken-pox. 'The only way I could console him was to let the rabbit stay in bed with him during the day,' his mother told the doctor. This made him prick up his ears since although he didn't know of any skin condition that could be transmitted from rabbits to humans the evidence was circumstantial and he asked Richard's mother to have Thumper checked. Just as in veterinary medicine it seems that for doctors too it is sometimes the parting, off-the-cuff remark which suddenly gives you the diagnosis!

So Richard, his anxious mum and his even more anxious rabbit were with me in my surgery. Anxious rabbits will suddenly buck, with no warning and tremendous force, with both hind legs as they try to jump away – for such small animals they have amazing convulsive strength. As soon as he was put on the table Thumper did the usual jumping about and eventually Richard was asked to be the nurse. In his hands the rabbit calmed down straight away. First I had a look at the boy's rash and, although I am not a human dermatologist, I immediately had an idea of the possible cause. I had seen many cases of dogs and cats infested with mites. The interesting and exciting thing was that I had never before seen human lesions like Richard's caused by a rabbit – probably because close contact, fur to skin, is much less common than it is with dogs and cats. I thought Richard's problem was probably down to a mite called *Cheyletiella*, which causes a skin rash and severe itching in humans. Animals show only mild symptoms of infestation, of which the most common is dandruff. In the rabbit *Cheyletiella* lives between the shoulder-blades and sure enough, slap between Thumper's shoulder-blades, was a patch of noticeable dandruff. Of course, this is something that just about everyone has from time to time and is generally ignored in a pet or treated with human shampoos, which have no effect on the likely causes. In Thumper's case, it had been noticed but as it was not apparently causing him any discomfort nothing had been done. I was quite excited: the chance was good of catching a mite and looking at it. All I had to do was pluck some hair and dandruff from between the rabbit's shoulder-blades, put it on a glass slide, put another slide on top, then search with the microscope.

Cheyletiella is one of the easiest mites to identify: it is just visible to the naked eye and, in heavy infestations, can be seen moving – which has led to the condition being called 'walking dandruff'. Under the microscope the mite is instantly recognizable: has large, nasty-looking hooks at its front end. This sight never fails to horrify people who have been bitten by it! Within a minute I had a perfect specimen in view and that was it. We had confirmed the cause of Thumper's dandruff, and almost certainly Richard's rash. It is always a good idea for owners to have a look at what has been biting them: it tends to concentrate their minds and ensure that treatment is thorough. Richard's mum was horrified to see the hugely magnified mite looking like something from a horror movie, although Richard seemed quite pleased!

As far as Richard was concerned the bad news was that Thumper was banned from his bed. Just that simple act, plus changing the bedding and spraying the bed would result in a cure for Richard. But what about his rabbit? Well, that wouldn't prove much of a problem either.

As the rabbit was so easy to handle – by other people, anyway – I elected to have him washed with an insecticide shampoo. The nurses did this right away, and a few hours later a shiny-clean Thumper was returned to his owner. First I had taken some photos for my collection but Richard was too embarrassed to show off his spots! Luckily I have other pictures of the characteristic rash that this mite produces and I am occasionally asked to show them to GPs. It's a great mite for getting vets and doctors together!

I wasn't always so quick to spot mite infestations. I saw my first case when I had been qualified all of three months and had only just been let loose on pets and their owners. I was predominantly a farm vet and filled in during evening surgeries. When Mrs Johnson brought her puppy in for vaccination I failed to notice that he had dandruff. Just as she was about to leave she said, 'Oh, by the way, do you think I should worry about his dandruff?' Years later I have come to regard those words, 'by the way', with extreme caution! Often owners will leave the thing that is really worrying them until the end, mentioning it almost as an afterthought. Failure to listen puts you in danger of missing the entire diagnosis – perhaps with disastrous consequences. My doctor friends tell me it's just the same with their patients. Anyway, on this occasion I wasn't listening and went along with her suggestion of using a human dandruff shampoo. About three weeks later, having forgotten about the puppy and Mrs Johnson, I was embarrassed to receive a call from Mrs Johnson's GP. He told me I should check her dog for a certain mite since his patient had typical lesions – he had found out that the family's pet had dandruff. Some months before, this GP had benefited from a lecture given by my boss so I felt even more humble, and my boss made sure of it.

The rest of the week settled down to routine work. Much of veterinary medicine in practice *is* mundane – vaccinations, castrations and spays – but the joy of it is that there is so much opportunity to learn even from common ailments. A good friend, an eminent doctor, put it another way: 'What you get out of your profession is equal to what you put in.'

One of the first operations I performed was for a condition so ordinary that I wonder why it is no more understood now than when I first qualified. I suppose this is because it is easily diagnosed, easily treated and tends to stay cured. The condition is aural haematoma, which means a blood blister in the ear. It's a perfect disease to study but has been mostly neglected. Usually the condition occurs when a dog or cat has another ear problem and continually shakes its head because of the irritation. Eventually a blood vessel bursts and the ear pinna fills with blood. The pet's response to this is to hang the head to one side, which, with a swollen ear, means that it is brought to the hospital.

And that brings me to a paradox: I often have a quiet moan to my clients for leaving things a bit late, but aural haematomas are best operated on after a week or so otherwise there's a risk of the blood reforming. The operation is quite simple: the ear is lanced, the blood, by now clotting nicely, is expressed and the pinna stitched together. If the operation is not done, the ear tends to collapse on itself leading to a 'cauliflower' ear. If you've ever seen a rough, tough tomcat, which has never had a proper home, you will probably have noticed his crumpled ears. It's not a pretty sight so we always operate on aural haematomas specifically to avoid this effect. It doesn't look pretty and a crumpled ear is prone to infections because of poor ventilation.

Jock, a middle-aged Scottish terrier, was a classic

example. (I wish, incidentally, that I had a pound for every Scottie I've met called Jock!). The poor chap had a real beauty. His right ear was swollen to three times its normal size and its sheer weight meant that when he wasn't shaking it he was walking around with his head at 45 degrees. Jock was a real toughie with other dogs and people, but fell to bits when confronted with the vet. I'm the same with doctors and dentists – and I know exactly why. It's fear of the needle. When I was about three I took my first trip to hospital – I'd fallen on some glass and cut my knee. All these years later I still have complete, vivid recall of my feelings and what happened in that casualty department. I can remember eyeing the sterilizers with dread as if I knew that they contained needles. Sure enough, the nurse produced one and stitched my knee. Each stitch – there were six in all – was proclaimed to be the last, and since then I have had a fear of needles!

I give countless injections every day, and every now and then I come across an animal with whom I empathize especially on account of our mutual fear. Jock was just such a dog. He began to tremble violently as soon as the nurse produced a syringe to give him his pre-anaesthetic sedative. Later as I came to give him the anaesthetic I noticed that his eyes were following me wherever I went and that as soon as I tried to inject him he panicked and tried to get off the table. I made a note on his card: 'Hates the sight of and feel of needles!' With this phobia I have found it best to conceal the needle so that the dog doesn't know it's going to get a jab.

Once Jock was asleep the operation proceeded smoothly and fifteen minutes later he was back in his cage. Later, before I went home I was passing Jock's cage so I opened the door and patted his head. His fear had gone: he wagged his tail as if he knew it was all over and he was going home soon.

Ten days later he was back. The ear had healed well, and as I was taking out the stitches I chatted to his owner, also known as Jock. He still had a strong Glaswegian accent in spite of living in London for fifty years. I asked Jock if he realised that his dog's fear of vets was connected to injections. Jock replied that it made sense although it hadn't occurred to him before. Apparently, some five years or so ago when he was a young dog, Jock had jumped when he was given his booster injection. Some of the vaccine had escaped so the injection had had to be repeated. The second attempt must have hit a nerve – this happens very rarely – and he let out a loud yell, then leaped off the table, bending the needle. The third, and successful, attempt needed two assistants to restrain him. His owner had forgotten about it – but not his dog! I suggested that we try to avoid injections for a while to see if we could desensitize Jock. The sight of his terrified eyes and shivering body was enough to stir pity in any vet's heart.

Some cases touch me more than others, and perhaps especially elderly animals. I suppose when I see pets with the illnesses associated with old age I am inevitably reminded of my own ageing – time seems to go so fast! Is it really thirty years since I emerged from college with my degree, faced with the daunting task of starting the real learning process? Old age, and the ailments peculiar to it, is a growth area in veterinary medicine now, and with the development of new drugs and techniques there is so much that can be done to lengthen pets' lives.

Spot was a sixteen-year-old mongrel suffering from a condition we see quite commonly in older dogs. He came into the hospital outpatient clinic one dismal February morning with a disease that any experienced vet would recognize instantly. But just as with Jock's aural

29

haematoma, we haven't advanced our understanding of it. Superficially Spot was a little like Jock in that his head was on one side – but there the resemblance ended. He had a severe head tilt and was hardly able to walk. When he tried, he staggered about and fell over. It had started quite suddenly at breakfast time and he had vomited. June, a widow in her seventies, was understandably worried

On the table I looked at his ears – no sign of any inflammation – but the real clue to the diagnosis was apparent as soon as I looked into Spot's eyes. The eyeballs were constantly flicking from side to side – a sign known as nystagmus. This is symptomatic of severe central-nervous-system derangement, and dogs with this condition are said to have suffered a 'stroke'. There is, however, no scientific evidence of a stroke in the human sense. In people, the cause is usually either a burst blood vessel or a blockage of a blood vessel in the brain. In dogs we lack any clear understanding as to why this dramatic and alarming symptom arises. It is sometimes called idiopathic vestibular syndrome, which means that although the problem arises in the brain we don't know the cause. The good news, though, is that most dogs make a good recovery, often within days.

'He's had a stroke, June,' I said, 'or, at least, the nearest equivalent to it that dogs can suffer.'

I looked up and saw tears in June's eyes. I thought I knew what she was thinking. 'Well, I know he's sixteen,' I went on, 'but there's no reason to give up just yet. You're not thinking of having him put to sleep, are you?'

'No, it's not that,' she replied, 'it's just that –,' and then she broke down completely. In between sobs she told me that her husband had died six months ago – of a stroke. I was immediately sorry that I had mentioned the dreaded word while I tried to comfort her. Apparently he and Spot had been inseparable since the dog was a puppy, and even now Spot would still sit by the front door waiting for his master to return, which June found almost unbearably sad. Maybe I should have said idiopathic vestibular disease but June wasn't the sort of person to be impressed by fancy-sounding conditions. Now, judging by her terrible distress, it was obvious that she thought Spot was going to go the same way as her husband.

'I don't think all's lost, June,' I said, trying to comfort her without being too optimistic – I couldn't be 100 per cent sure at Spot's advanced age that he would recover, although I felt there was a good chance he'd get over it. 'Let me have him in the hospital a few days. There's no harm in trying.'

June agreed and said a tearful goodbye to Spot, who was taken down to the prep room, put on a drip and given light sedation to prevent the vomiting, caused by the dizzy feel-ing induced in its turn by the constant movement of his eyes. It must be worse than any fairground ride. There's no evidence that any particular treatment is beneficial but I usually give antibiotics, in case there's any infection, and steroids, to reduce any possible inflammation in the brain. Over the years I've seen friends and colleagues try many different treatments, but I think Nature usually sorts this one out, provided that you give support in the form of drips and symptomatic treatment.

Sure enough, two days later on ward rounds, I was happy to see Spot tucking into his breakfast. He had stopped vomiting, the nystagmus had gone, and he was able to walk properly. I telephoned June myself and told her to come and pick up her dog as soon as she could as he wanted to go home. Her joy brought a lump to my throat. It's so nice to give a dog a lease of life when the owner isn't expecting it. When June came in I explained that Spot still had his head tilt and that this might not improve completely, but otherwise a full recovery was now on the cards. The best of it is that attacks like this are often one-offs.

A tilted head can also be a sign of inner-ear disease, or *otitis interna* to give it its medical name. It occurs when the ear drum ruptures Usually there is obvious involvement of the ear although sometimes it's necessary to anaesthetize the dog, then to look inside the ears and take X-rays to make the diagnosis. Many dogs can only be cured by complicated surgery. But while I have seen hundreds of inner-ear diseases in dogs I had never seen one in a mouse until about ten minutes after June had departed with Spot.

The last patient of the afternoon session had a pronounced head tilt. John Brooks had brought in his ten-year-old daughter Lesley's mouse. He had recently lost his job and, with time on his hands, he was happy to bring Lesley's pet to the clinic. Pretty soon, however, I found that – as is usual when the actual owner isn't present – it was almost impossible to get a clear history of the animal. Poor John knew nothing about this mouse, not even its sex! However, it had a head tilt, which suggested inner-ear disease so I started off with an injection of antibiotic and asked John if he could get permission from Lesley's teacher for her to have the next afternoon off school.

The next day John was back with an anxious Lesley, who was full of information. Normally I start by checking the diet: everything was correct – good-quality commercial mouse pellets with a little fruit, vegetables and, amusingly, the occasional dog biscuit to which the mouse (called George) was apparently addicted. At two he was getting on a bit (between two and three years is the normal mouse lifespan). His head tilt had come on suddenly two days before and he was a little bit under the weather. With Lesley's help

I was able to get a look at his ear, which was infected. It was, indeed, inner-ear disease and carried a poor outlook. Lesley, though, was nothing if not an optimist and maintained that there had been progress even in the last twenty-four hours. There's simply no way of telling, especially with these little creatures, what will happen and sometimes, with dedication and the right antibiotic, miracles can happen. Dedication was something Lesley had in abundance and, armed with a syringe and antibiotic syrup, which she would make sure got into George's stomach, she left, with her bemused dad trailing behind her. I kept my fingers crossed.

Although it was February the mild weather continued. Ever the pessimist, I thought that if this were to last there would be a fantastic flea epidemic in the summer. We were already seeing an unusually high number of skin-disease cases caused by fleas. If this is truly global warming it's only a matter of time before we start to see tropical diseases in Britain. Countries just two hours away by plane have numerous weird and wonderful diseases, such as heart worm – transmitted by mosquitoes – and another one currently seen in Spain, Italy and Greece called Leishmaniasis which is transmitted by sand flies Could these get a hold in the UK if our climate continues to warm up?

The next day Richard and Thumper were back for a check-up. Richard's rash had cleared up and, to his joy, he had scored a hat trick in a school football match. Like most of the kids who live near the hospital, he was an Arsenal supporter and modelled himself on Ian Wright, the prolific goal-scorer. His ambition was to play for the Gunners. Thumper was doing splendidly. Richard and his mum had bathed him once more and there wasn't a trace of dandruff, either between his shoulder-blades or anywhere else. I looked carefully with a magnifying glass and, after a few minutes, was happy to pronounce him cured He had been banished from the bed and Richard had accepted this, the compromise being that Thumper was staying in his room in a cardboard box at night. I received a letter from his doctor, saying how pleased he was that by collaboration between us a diagnosis had been made. He sounded as pleased as I was!

Towards the end of the month I was confronted with an unusual emergency. Postmen will tell you that dogs can inflict nasty bites and are frequently hostile to anyone in uniform. The most dangerous moment for a postman comes when he puts his hand through the letterbox. Some dogs will wait quietly by the door and try to bite the hand, others bark furiously as soon as they hear footsteps on the path. Bonzo was a black and white mongrel, not much bigger than a Jack Russell terrier, who lived in a first-floor maisonette. At the first hint of the postman's arrival he would charge down a flight of twenty stairs in an attempt to get at the intruder At twelve, he was a bit long in the tooth for this athletic activity. Not only that, but he was rather podgy too. He had always been very protective of his home – which was welcomed by Bob and Judy Jackson, his pensioner owners – and they learned to introduce him to any visitors, telling him they were friends. They had tried to do this without success with various postmen over the years. It's funny how some dogs just take a dislike to certain people and nothing will change it.

On this occasion Bonzo had crashed down the full flight of stairs, ending up in a heap at the bottom and colliding with a pushchair belonging to the neighbours. He had lost consciousness for five minutes and was only semi-conscious when Bob and Judy got him into the hospital. It was clear that Bob and Judy Jackson were terribly upset. Bonzo was very much their child and this accident was a terrible disaster for them both. Bonzo remained semi-conscious for two days, needing constant drips and shock treatment. We diagnosed severe concussion and it took more than a week before he began to make slow progress. After three days he could stand up. A day later he could walk but only in circles and was completely disoriented. At the end of the week he was still subdued. I was worried that he had suffered permanent brain damage but felt that he was well enough to be sent home, with a guarded outlook for complete recovery.

I was pleased to see him again a few days later, more or less back to normal. Bob and Judy told me that he had undergone a complete personality change: he was much more relaxed about everything, he hardly barked at all and greeted everyone who visited them as a long-lost friend. Previously he had had to be shut up in the spare room before a stranger could be let in. Even the postman had elicited a wag! I can only assume that the shock of the accident had caused a temporary loss of blood to the brain, which had had this effect on Bonzo. In all other respects he was his old self, so Bob and Judy were in a way quite pleased that he had calmed down, although they were still a bit shaky having nearly lost their dog.

I had never seen anything like Bonzo's case before and in a way it seemed typical of the month, which had been pretty unusual anyway with the weather so mild. I had seen things I hadn't seen before, and others that had reminded me of how little I know even as an experienced vet. In another month it would be time for the annual congress of the British Small Animal Veterinary Association – I must remember to write down all the puzzling cases and look for the answers then.

MARCH

March is never my favourite month. By now most people are fed up with winter, and yet it may be another two months before the onset of warm, sunny weather A few years ago this was the month in which I went skiing but with a young family I have temporarily put ski holidays on hold and look forward instead to the summer.

So much the better, then, at the beginning of the month, to have a potentially devastating case, which was – thank goodness – simple to deal with. From the look on her face, Bella's owner was at her wit's end. After a few years in practice most vets can pick up the 'vibes' from their clients as soon as they walk through the door: often they have decided that it is time for their pet to be put to sleep and just want reassurance that they have made the correct decision. At other times, they are fearful that this will be the vet's advice and may burst into tears of relief when they find out that this won't be necessary.

Bella wasn't ill as such: rather, her problem was making life unbearable for her family. She didn't seem able to control her bladder any more, especially when she was asleep. Jackie, a single parent with two daughters aged eleven and ten, had first assumed it was down to old age (Bella was fifteen) and had tried hard to solve the problem. Putting newspapers everywhere had helped at first and later blankets, although this became a nuisance with the washing-machine constantly on the go. Gradually Jackie became worn down and the flat began to smell as she couldn't keep up with Bella's chronic urine dribble. Eventually she decided to seek help from a vet, even though friends had told her she should 'get the dog put down'.

As I was quick to reassure Jackie, incontinence in old dogs is quite common and often treatable. Looking at Bella, a beautiful black Labrador, as she sat placidly on the consulting-room table there didn't seem to be much wrong with her. From what Jackie had told me she was very well, eating and drinking normally. She hadn't lost weight, but wasn't fat either, and was her bright, cheerful self. Obviously, at fifteen, she no longer felt inclined to dash about like a two-year-old, but still liked to chase the odd squirrel or pigeon in the park – just to show she wasn't past it! All in all she was in magnificent condition.

Jackie had brought in a urine specimen, which Bella had obligingly provided outside the hospital. Getting a urine sample from a dog, male or female, is surprisingly easy. For a bitch I usually suggest putting a flat tray under the dog when she squats; only a little is required and this can be transferred into a bottle. Then we dip a special strip of paper into the specimen, watch the paper change colour, then compare it with the colour-code on the container of the strips. A surprising amount of information is provided within a minute. In Bella's case all was normal, which meant that diabetes, kidney or bladder infections were unlikely. In an old animal, like Bella, it was much more likely that the sphincter that controls urination had weakened and was unable to prevent leaking, especially when she was lying down or when she jumped up or did anything that increased pressure on her tummy muscles. Nevertheless I did some blood tests to confirm that disease was absent and to make sure Bella's liver was functioning.

The next day I was passing on the hopeful news to Jackie that everything was apparently normal.

'We've got a drug that might help Bella,' I said. 'You will have to put some drops into her food every day and with a bit of luck that will tighten up the control of the bladder.' Jackie looked doubtful. After all, it was only yesterday that she had come to the hospital expecting the worst and coming to terms with the fact that she would be going home alone. 'Let's give it a couple of weeks,' I added. 'We can start to worry if there's no improvement by then.'

As they left the consulting room I crossed my fingers. Watching Bella bounce out, wagging her tail furiously in the way that dogs do when they are leaving the surgery, I felt sure that her time hadn't come yet and I found myself looking forward to seeing them again.

We take it for granted living with a pet is always going to be easy, especially when we have enjoyed years of harmonious co-existence, so it comes as a shock when problems like incontinence rapidly destroy the peace. My next patient after Bella was also causing his owner inconvenience. Mick was a lively two-year-old yellow Labrador, and his owner was a widower called Michael. Mick's breath smelt awful, which was obvious as soon as he had been in the room for a few minutes! Michael was keen to talk about his own diagnosis, which was bad teeth, and wanted to know when I could 'fix them' so that his grandchildren would start visiting again. His daughter-in-law had put her foot down once the smell had become unbearable. Mick's teeth, however, were white and healthy and I soon pointed out to his owner where the real problem was.

'It's usually spaniels who get this,' I said, 'but smell this!' I had found deep folds of infected skin along the dog's lips. I put a swab of cotton wool in the crack and then held it to Michael's nose. He recoiled in horror and came out with a couple of words I won't repeat here! Mick had abnormal folds of skin along his lips, which had become wet with saliva. In this damp, poorly ventilated area infection was near certainty and the undoubted cause of the smell. The solution would be a relatively simple operation to cut out the folds, a basic form of plastic surgery, and I found a slot on the next day's operating list.

Even though it wasn't cold by normal standards for March, it was chilly enough, but there was no alternative to opening the windows wide in the prep room the next day when I gave Mick an anaesthetic and prepared him for his operation. After clipping away the hair from the affected skin the extent of the problem was clear. Poor Mick must have been suffering because the skin under his lips was very inflamed. He had not shown much sign of this apart from rubbing his mouth on the carpet – which, of course, had made things even worse for the house. All I had to do was cut out the inflamed skin and the fold. Years ago when I first did this I was alarmed by the amount of blood that welled up in the operating site, and I used to spend ages trying to pick off every leaking blood vessel. Later, I discovered that the small ones would automatically seal once the skin was stitched back together. The area round the lips is abundantly supplied with blood, which makes for rapid and usually uneventful healing.

Three-quarters of an hour later Mick was coughing out the tube that connected his lungs to the anaesthetic machine. Instead of sore, smelly lips he now had two lines of stitches in healthy skin. The smell had gone. He would need an Elizabethan-style ruff collar round his neck to stop him scratching at his lips while the healing was going on but he could go home later that day. I was looking forward to seeing him in ten days to take the stitches out.

This is the joy of surgery – the results are there to see quite quickly. Medical cases bring a different sort of satisfaction from trying to puzzle out what is going on and using the right tests to find out. The downside of surgery is the unfortunate truth that not every operation is successful and surgeons have to learn from those cases that don't go well.

Another of the joys of being a veterinary surgeon is that there is an unlimited number of diseases and conditions to learn about. In recent years the Royal College of Veterinary Surgeons has encouraged the study of specialist subjects by creating new postgraduate courses. Each certificate needs two or three years of intensive study and there's no doubt in my mind that this has led to an explosion of knowledge, with thousands of vets raising their own standards in many areas – one of which is veterinary dentistry and many practices can now offer quite advanced techniques to preserve teeth.

Fifi, a miniature poodle, had a well-recognized dental problem, which was challenging but didn't need specialist help. She had been seen by Helen in her clinic one afternoon in February with a discharging abscess under the eye. In these cases, the abscess develops in a sinus behind a large tooth in the upper jaw called the carnassial tooth. The sinus, which is just a big space, is called the malar sinus and the abscess, not surprisingly, the malar abscess. The problem with these abscesses is that they cannot drain because the tooth is in the way so they erupt from under the eye. But drainage from here is never 100 per cent so the abscess doesn't heal. Fifi was a rather ancient sixteen-year-old and Helen was reluctant to book her in for an operation to remove the tooth on two counts: first, because of the anaesthetic risk, and second, because Fifi's jaw was fragile and might break if the tooth was taken out. A full course of antibiotics hadn't resolved the problem, and now the abscess had caused the skin under the eye to become inflamed. Fifi was experiencing significant discomfort. We would have to operate. Fifi's owner, Mrs Jenkins, was a sprightly old lady in her eighties and, although worried, put a brave face on it.

During the morning session Helen and I were in the prep room together; as she was fixing a broken leg I opted to sort out Fifi. The first hurdle was the anaesthetic. I wasn't too worried as we had done a full blood screen and, for her age, Fifi seemed remarkably healthy. In any case, the anaesthetics we use now are as safe as possible and are, in fact, similar to those used in human hospitals. Fifi's teeth turned out to be in a fearful state and one by one I gently levered them out, including the carnassial that had caused the abscess. Finally, there was just one diseased tooth left in the lower jaw. I extracted it carefully. Suddenly there was a quiet crack as the jaw under it split in two. This was my worst fear and I cursed under my breath. Just then Helen popped over to see how I was getting on. She was still scrubbed up as she had just finished her operation.

'Look what's happened to this one,' I said. 'It's your miniature poodle case.'

Helen cast an eye over the jaw and felt inside Fifi's mouth. 'I reckon I can fix that,' she announced.

Thank heavens for colleagues! I was upset that things had gone wrong, but then watched Helen and helped as she deftly introduced a small steel pin along the length of Fifi's lower jaw. The end result was a perfectly firm and stable jaw. I was very grateful to her, and over coffee we discussed how to avoid this mishap. With difficulty, it seemed, although a similar thing had happened to Helen once

42

before, which was why she had been so quick to remedy the situation. But it had given me a fright and reminded me, as if I needed reminding, that surgical cases don't always go to plan and also, of course, of the universal truth that two heads are better than one! The next day, on ward rounds, I was happy to see Fifi eating soft food without difficulty.

That night, while I was on duty, I saw another old dog and his aged owner. The old man had come in with his granddaughter and Rex, a small mongrel, who had obviously come to the end of a long life. He had been poorly for a few days but over the last few hours had taken a turn for the worse. He was lying down, very sleepy, and couldn't be roused. It was as if he had decided that he had lived long enough. I checked him over and he had many of the signs of kidney failure. His breath had a strong ammonia-like smell and he had not eaten for two days. Today he had started to vomit. For about a month previously he had been drinking more than usual and losing weight. Looking at him now, unable to stand and breathing shallowly, it was obvious that he needed a helping hand to pass away peacefully.

'How old is he?' I asked Bert, his owner.

'I've had him since he was a pup – twenty-two years.'

'That's a good age by any standards, and you've done him proud, but I think he's failing fast.'

Bert nodded, but I could tell that he had expected this. His granddaughter spoke now. 'We've all been expecting the end for some time, with the dog being so old. My granddad's ninety-nine, by the way.'

I glanced at Bert in astonishment – he looked in his seventies. I said to him, as gently as I could, 'I think it's time to let Rex go.' I have had to give this advice week in week out through all my career but it never gets any easier. Poor Bert turned his back to me and I could see by the shake of his shoulders that he had started to cry. His granddaughter comforted him, but I felt a lump in my throat too, at the thought of the many happy hours that the old man and his dog had spent together. Rex, though, was deteriorating by the minute so, with Bert holding him, I injected the barbiturate into his vein and he slipped peacefully away with a last sigh.

After stroking Rex's head for the last time, Bert and his granddaughter had a sit-down in the waiting room while they waited to be picked up. Meanwhile I finished off the emergency clinic and joined them later. I was relieved to see that Bert had brightened up.

'Do you have any other pets?' I asked him.

'I've got another dog,' he replied. 'He's seventeen!'

I had to ask him how he had managed to live so long and so well himself, and seemingly ensured the same for his pets. 'Simple,' said Bert, with a twinkle in his eye. 'You just have to get up every day at six in the morning.'

'And he does,' added his granddaughter, with pride.

'Well, that dashes my hopes,' I said. 'Getting up that early was never my strong point.'

As they left I couldn't but admire Bert's spirit and obvious zest for life and hoped he would enjoy many more years in spite of his age. I overheard his granddaughter telling him that the family would make sure that he would always have a dog. And it would be a lucky dog too.

The next day the unseasonably mild weather continued. At this rate the year would go down as virtually free of the miseries of winter. Soon the clocks would go forward and the lighter evenings would dispel the gloom. After Easter we would have to gear ourselves up for the increased workload of the warmer months. . .

I was reminded of Easter again the next day when we

had a most unlikely patient for an inner-London small-animal hospital. It was a black lamb, which had been found under very strange circumstances. Somebody had spotted some children playing with it on a train in the East End of London. When asked by the transport police the children denied all knowledge of the lamb or how it had got on to the train. At most it was only a week old and should have been with its mother. The lamb was transported to the Harmsworth and all the nurses immediately fell in love with it. The first hurdle was getting the little creature to learn to suck from a bottle. After several attempts it got the message and then proceeded to demolish all the milk it could. There was much competition as to who should feed the lamb. Meanwhile the hunt was on for the owner and we persuaded some contacts in Kent to foster the lamb on a farm. Several of the nurses had photographs taken with the lamb and we were sorry to see her go the following weekend. It never ceased to amaze me that, no matter what animal turns up, we can usually find someone to care for it!

The following Monday Bella was back with Jackie. As they walked in I knew that the drops were working. Jackie wore a broad smile and the penetrating smell of urine from the dog was gone. The treatment had started to work almost immediately and a thorough spring clean had freshened up the home. Jackie's two young daughters were especially pleased since they had grown up with Bella and couldn't imagine life without her. Bella would have to have the drops in her food for the rest of her life but everyone could live with that!

Also, as I had expected, Mick's operation had been a success. There he was, a few hours later, held on the table by Michael while I set about removing the stitches. Healing had been perfect and Mick's mouth now looked clean and dry. His demeanour had changed too: Labradors are usually placid and gentle but he had become more content and at ease now that the irritation had gone. The news of his cure had travelled fast and the grandchildren were visiting again – another thing that made the dog happy. Michael was almost beside himself with gratitude but he needn't have thanked me – just being able to be comfortably in the same room and seeing the complete absence of any inflammation around the lips was thanks enough. This was a good start to the week and, as so often happens, things continued in that vein – at least for a while.

We had had a spate of poisoning cases in the hospital during the last week, in some cats and a dog. The cats had been suspected of eating alpha chloralose, in rodent bait. It's sometimes difficult to prove but the symptoms are classic. Cats usually come in with tremendous trembling and shaking, and are unable to stand. Pretty soon their temperature drops and keeping them warm is an important part of the treatment. It has an alarming appearance but the good news is that, with quick action, most are saved. One cat had come in over the weekend in a fairly bad way. Bairbre, the vet on duty, had put up a drip, wrapped her in warm blankets with a hot-water bottle and instructed the nurses to observe her over the next twenty-four hours and make sure the drip kept flowing. The next morning on ward rounds the cat, a much-loved tabby called Dilly, was responding well to treatment and would probably be able to go home in a day or so. Once these poison cases start to get better progress is usually rapid; all that is required is supportive treatment and the body does the rest. The liver is the main detoxification organ and, in young animals like Dilly, it is effective.

Also over that weekend – Bairbre had been kept busy – was a dog that had swallowed some rat poison containing

Warfarin, which causes massive internal bleeding unless caught quickly. The Boxer, whose name was Rocky, had been brought in as soon as his distraught owners had seen him swallow the poison granules. Typically he was under a year old, when dogs, like young children, get up to all sorts of mischief. Bairbre had given him some washing-soda crystals, which made Rocky very sick indeed. In the vomit the blue Warfarin crystals could be seen but, just to be sure, he was also given vitamin K, an antidote for this class of poison. It had all been successful because, on checking Rocky the next day, he had a lovely healthy colour with no sign of bleeding. Accidental poisoning is such a tragedy, often involves young animals and causes such anguish that it is fantastic when the animals involved can be saved.

Another common tragedy that affects cats and dogs is the road accident. With dogs, I believe that virtually all are avoidable: it's just a question of ensuring that the dog is under control on a lead whenever there is any chance of coming into contact with cars. Over the years I have gained the impression that accidents in owned dogs are fewer but we see many strays with broken limbs after a run-in with a car. With cats, it's difficult to know how to prevent such accidents, except to keep them in if there are dangerous busy roads nearby.

Fluffy was a typical example of what I see almost daily. A young – just under a year old – tomcat, not yet neutered, he had come into the emergency weekend surgery, having presumably been run over by a car. He had managed to get home but was lame on one of his back legs. When he was fit he would need an X-ray. On the Monday morning I was on the X-ray rota, which we all share, and there in front of me, looking sorry for himself, was Fluffy. His shock symptoms had been stabilized and he had been kept reasonably free from pain with injections, but he was still pretty uncomfortable.

A minute later he was fast asleep under the anaesthetic while I positioned him for the X-ray. I had had a gentle feel while he was still conscious and discovered that the pain was around his hip. This meant one of three common possibilities, of which the most likely was a break at the top of the thigh bone just below the hip joint. However, his leg might be dislocated or his pelvis broken. I sat watching him while Lisa, my nurse for the morning session, developed the X-ray.

Two minutes later we had our answer: a fracture at the top of the thigh bone. The standard procedure for this is to remove the whole of the top of the femur, or the femoral head, as it is usually called. This is effectively half the hip joint and we rely on Nature's healing process to form a fibrous false joint over the next couple of months. Although at first sight this is a rather brutal operation, cats seem to make a rapid recovery and need no further treatment after the stitches are taken out. I decided to go ahead with the 'excision arthroplasty'. All that is required is to cut down to the head of the thigh bone where it is broken, then remove it. Having discussed it with his owner, Bob, the next thing to do for Fluffy was to castrate him: wandering too far afield in search of female cats had probably been the root cause of his accident. From now on, he would be more home loving and less inclined to roam. An injection of painkiller and antibiotic and he was back in his cage, coming round and soon looking a lot more comfortable.

On the last day of the month I had an unusual patient to deal with: a pipistrelle bat. This is the smallest of the British bats and, although widespread in London, I can remember seeing only a couple in the hospital. This one had been picked up in an exhausted state near to an inner-city church. It was tiny, weighing only about 3.5 grams, which is quite a bit underweight. Normally these bats weigh 5–6 grams and have a wing span of 22 centimetres. Although not much is known about diseases in them we were unable to find much that was physically wrong and suspected that it had come out of hibernation and become weak from lack of food. The end of March is the usual time for bats to wake up and we had had a warmish couple of days followed almost immediately by a brief cold snap. For a few days it was touch and go for the bat but several of the nurses, especially Clare, who is keen on all aspects of wildlife, had persevered with the little creature. They had managed to get him to eat and as I went into ward eight I saw him tucking into a mealworm held for him by Clare. In an amazingly short time he had put on weight and now tipped the scales at 6 grams. Hopes were high of releasing him back into the colony near the church, probably in the next few days when we could be reasonably sure of his survival.

What a month it had been! Everything from a lamb to dogs with halitosis and incontinence to run-over or poisoned cats. And a bat. By and large it had been a successful and fulfilling month and now, even though it was cold and snowing up north, spring was around the corner.

APRIL

April continued cold, which kept patient numbers down. This was fortunate because within a few days most of the vets were at the annual congress for small-animal veterinary surgeons, held at the state-of-the-art congress centre in Birmingham. A volunteer had had to stand in for weekend duty while the rest of us enjoyed a tremendous get-together of over six thousand vets. This year Helen stayed behind to hold the fort.

Keeping up-to-date is a phenomenal task and we all try to get to at least five days of 'continuing professional development' (CPD) each year. Many congresses are held both at home and abroad, also weekend and day courses, and it becomes a problem to fit them all in. Another problem for me and many others is to decide which lectures to go to at the main congress in Birmingham. At any time five or six are in session – it's easy to become saturated with knowledge and get very tired. One of the great things, though, is catching up with friends, colleagues and classmates from years ago: there's always a good social programme, and lots of vets make it a family occasion.

Ideally, the following Monday we should all be back at work full of new ideas and enthusiasm, although the reality is that we usually need a few days to get over the congress.

One of my first cases in the Monday afternoon clinic following the congress involved something that crops up commonly at this time of year. Ulysses, a male tortoise of at least forty years old, had come out of hibernation a few weeks ago – rather early for him. Every year for as long as his owner, Ann, had kept him, he would wake up on 5 April, which was easy to remember as it was also her daughter's birthday. This year, however, he had woken up during a spell of mild weather and had been unwell ever since. He had not eaten a thing, which was most unusual since he loved his food. All sorts of vegetables, cucumber, cabbage and even imported strawberries had failed to tempt him. Most tortoises we see in this state in April turn out to have post-hibernation anorexia, which just means that they fail to eat after waking up. During hibernation the tortoise lives on the fat reserves it has accumulated during the previous summer. If they run down to a low level before the end of hibernation the body protein provides energy. Then if the tortoise wakes too soon and doesn't begin eating he can become ill. Ulysses was a classic example of this and would need treatment in hospital.

First he was measured and weighed. The results were recorded on a graph and we learned that Ulysses' weight was dangerously low for his length, and that he would need fluids and feeding by stomach tube plus multivitamin injections to build him up. Also the nurses would give him warm baths every day. He would have blood tests to check liver and kidney function: from these we would find out if, and how badly, he was dehydrated.

The next day on ward rounds, there was Sam, his nurse, feeding him by stomach tube with special easily digested food and water-replacement solution.

A few days later I was due in court – and couldn't help reflecting on the devotion and hard work being lavished on Ulysses in comparison with the sad story that unfolded now. Ben, a German shepherd dog, had been presented to me by Inspector John Bowe some months before. Ben was the subject of a cruelty complaint by a member of the public. A dog had been heard barking constantly but never seen, and the person who alerted the RSPCA was worried that the dog might be suffering. When the inspectors arrived, they discovered a large dog in a cellar. Anyone passing would cause it to bark. No one was in the house and after a while the police were called to break into the cellar. This was relatively simple and the RSPCA inspector cautiously went in. In spite of the ferocious noise, Ben turned out to be a nice, friendly dog and was brought into the hospital for examination. But the conditions inside the cellar shocked the inspectors and the police: there was no light, the floor was littered with sheep bones, the smell was dreadful and it was filthy beyond description.

When Ben was removed from his 'home', he blinked in the unaccustomed light and appeared bewildered and excitable. Back at the hospital he was difficult to examine, barking and whining and jumping about. With the aid of a sedative injection I was able to get a good look at him. His coat was smelly and very dirty. At first sight he seemed overweight but the shocking thing was that when I came to examine his muscle mass I found it virtually non-existent. I could only think that the dog had not exercised – and therefore not used his muscles – for some considerable time. His claws confirmed this: they were shockingly overgrown. This alone would be enough for a cruelty prosecution since the poor dog couldn't walk without considerable pain. I had estimated that he had suffered for at least three months and this was the basis of the prosecution case.

As the depressing details of Ben's experience were recounted in court I was impressed as always by how thorough the process was. My part was quite simple: I had to

53

state my findings on the day of my examination of the dog. Graphic photographs of his conditions were displayed to the magistrates. But it wasn't this evidence that was the eye opener for me. All the circumstances were gone into in great detail – and for the first time in a long time I was shocked too. . .

For Ben's owner the sorry state of affairs had been precipitated by the death of her husband. For the first time ever she had found herself alone, without the support of her grown-up family. It seemed a good idea to keep the dog: the area was known for burglary and Ben would provide security. Within a short space of time, though, she hadn't been able to manage him. He was too big and she wasn't able to control him when out for walks. No one seemed interested in helping her. She made a few attempts to re-home him then gave up. Ben stayed where he was in the cellar with food thrown in but exercise stopped – *for three years*. This is what shocked me. No wonder he had been so excited when he came out.

Ben's owner was found guilty of causing unnecessary suffering and the magistrates imposed a substantial fine with costs but not a ban on keeping dogs. They have the power to ban people for life from keeping a pet and this, for me, is the best solution in most of these cases. Prevention of cruelty is assured by the application of that punishment, and people have long memories so there are no worries about it being forgotten. As for Ben, he was re-homed almost immediately after the court case to a lovely family where he is doing well, apparently having forgiven and forgotten his three years' imprisonment.

The next day I saw a dog that looked just like Ben – it was uncanny – but his owner couldn't have been more concerned for his welfare. In fact, she was in tears. Mrs Beck

54

was middle-aged, with an invalid husband, and her dog, Sabre, was very much one of the family. He was a great companion for her housebound husband when she was out. For four days Sabre had been limping on one of his back legs and it was getting worse. Mrs Beck had been walking him in the park when she met another German shepherd owner, who reckoned that the dog probably had hip dysplasia. Not surprisingly, this on-the-spot diagnosis frightened her. Hip dysplasia is a fairly common problem in various breeds of dog, although many breeders are taking active measures to reduce its incidence by careful screening programmes. It is a congenital defect of the hips, in which the hips are effectively too shallow. Later in life, affected dogs will suffer varying degrees of lameness and arthritis. The other owner had told Mrs Beck that she had had to have a dog put down on account of the same condition.

There she was then with Sabre expecting me to confirm her worse fears or at best tell her that the dog would have to be put down sooner rather than later. The only way hip dysplasia or arthritis can be confirmed is by taking an X-ray, which would need a general anaesthetic. I didn't want to rush into this as Sabre was twelve, which is getting on a bit for a German shepherd. Mrs Beck walked him round the consulting table and the limping was plain to see. Now I had to check out where the pain was coming from. As soon as I went anywhere near his back legs Sabre started to get nasty, with much snarling and growling – but at least he gave me adequate warning. Earlier that day I had had a narrow miss with a dog that wagged his tail then snapped without any warning.

'He wasn't like this with the last vet!' said Mrs Beck.

I grimaced. 'Perhaps he wasn't in so much pain last time,' I said, remembering that if the dog doesn't like you

55

the owner sometimes won't either. On the, fortunately rare, occasions that I have been bitten, the owner has always maintained, 'That's the first time he's ever done that!'

A muzzle on Sabre's snout gave me the confidence I needed to get on with a proper examination. This did not go down well with Mrs Beck, though. I tried to explain that I needed to be certain where the pain in the leg was coming from so that if an X-ray was needed we would centre on the right place, but I felt I was fighting a losing battle for her good opinion.

The most obvious thing right from the start was that Sabre was feeling no obvious pain in his hips. I moved down his leg, finding nothing until I got near the paws. Then it became apparent where the problem was: there was a large infected cut on one of the pads, which was inflamed and painful. I had a careful look, but there was nothing in it. Sabre had probably trodden on some glass while out for a walk. Ten days of antibiotics should clear the infection and cure his limp. Mrs Beck's reaction to this good news was to burst into tears. It just doesn't pay to listen to what other dog owners tell you, especially if the advice is alarming.

As I opened the consulting-room door to see Mrs Beck out, I heard a familiar voice holding forth in the waiting room, advising on the treatment of fleas with herbs. It was Mrs Fortuna, an elderly lady who, in spite of her name, was English. I had never heard her speak of a husband so I had assumed she was a widow. She had a lot of cats as pets, and one dog, the long-suffering Mr Harry. A frequent visitor, she had been in today to see Stan with him. She had read about ear mites in dogs and cats and because the dog had shaken his head a few times she was worried he had them. After an exhaustive search Stan had found nothing wrong and therefore prescribed nothing.

Now Mr Harry was sitting in the corridor, looking rather bored and waiting patiently to go home, while his owner went up the lines of people waiting, dishing out her own brand of remedies – she had some advice for just about everything, not to mention a 'thing' about tinned dog food. Most of the owners seemed to enjoy chatting to her – pets are a great icebreaker – but I never knew if her advice was ever taken.

'It looks like we're going to have a downpour,' I said, in passing to her. 'Don't let Mr Harry get caught in it – he'll get pneumonia.' This was to remind her gently to get on her way and stop worrying the life out of the rest of the afternoon's patients!

Of these, Butch seemed, to his owner, the victim of old age. Formerly a strapping terrier-cross he had become fat and was losing his hair. Worse, he had developed a pot belly and was drinking lots of water. His owners, a retired couple, hadn't thought about consulting the vet as Butch was thirteen, after all. As soon as I saw him, though, I had a pretty shrewd idea as to what might be wrong with him. On talking to his owners, Mr and Mrs Cooper, I found out that he had a real drinking problem. He was getting through about eight pints of water a day. Worse, he was getting his owners up every night to go out to spend a penny.

'Why didn't you come to see us earlier?' I said. I felt so sorry for them, getting up night after night – with a young family I know full well how exhausting that is! Butch's pot-belly was due to an enlarged liver, which I could easily feel. All his muscles were wasting, which added to the pot-bellied appearance since his tummy muscles couldn't support the weight of his liver. His skin was very thin – I could see the blood vessels through it. With the hair loss he had the classic signs of a disease called Cushing's syndrome.

57

Before the arrival of Gabriel on the veterinary team, I would have said that this was a relatively rare condition in dogs, but it turned out that Gabriel had an amazing talent for diagnosing it: within six months of him joining us we had had quite a number of cases. I don't think the rest of us were missing them, it was just that Gabriel picked them up right from the start.

Cushing's syndrome is caused by the adrenal glands enlarging and producing too much cortisone, which causes all the symptoms. Most cases are sparked off by minute cancers in a part of the brain called the pituitary gland and a smaller number are caused by cancer of the adrenal gland itself. The diagnosis rests on taking blood tests during the day, to measure the levels of cortisone in the blood. These are sent off to an outside laboratory and the results are generally available within a week. If my diagnosis was confirmed there was a treatment that would give Butch a good chance of a normal life and a return to a more youthful appearance – not to mention a resumption of good sleep for his owners. We would have to wait and see.

April is the month when we see large numbers of ducklings in the hospital. We can have up to a dozen at a time, occasionally more. A large heat-lamp serves as Mum and the ducklings spend most of their time basking under it. We provide them with food, shelter and warmth until we move them on to specialist centres for rearing. Generally they do very well, with the majority going on to be released successfully. One morning when I caught sight of Kieran Graham, the ambulance driver, leaving us with another batch I made a mental note to ask him why we see so many at this time of the year.

As it happened I bumped into him a few days later in the Crown Court. He had been involved in the rescue of four adult dogs and three pups, which had been left in a dilapidated wreck of a car without food or water. The RSPCA had been called out and, with the assistance of the police, the car was broken into and the dogs brought to the hospital. Except for one pup, they were emaciated and had lice. The conditions inside the car had been appalling. This had happened over a year ago, and the person responsible had taken some tracking down, but eventually the case had been heard at the magistrates' court where the dogs' owner, a Mr L, had elected to defend himself. The essence of our case had been that these dogs had been abandoned in a situation likely to cause them suffering and that, being so emaciated, they had been inadequately cared for. The four adult dogs were subsequently to increase their weight by up to 40 per cent just by being fed without any other treatment. In other words they were not ill as such, just starving. Halfway through the proceedings Mr L had fallen out with the magistrates and the case had continued without him. He had been found guilty, sent to prison, and banned from keeping dogs for ten years. As far as I was concerned, this was a just result and I was happy with it. I looked forward to seeing the dogs in caring homes. Mr L, however, had other ideas and wanted them back. He simply would not accept that he had caused them suffering and appealed against the decision. So that's why Kieran and I were outside the court waiting for the case to be heard, this time with a judge presiding.

I asked Kieran about the latest ducklings. He told me that they were usually, as in this case, mallards and the problem was almost always due to the ducks nesting in dangerous locations such as at the top of high-rise buildings on balconies. As the ducklings grew they invariably fell out of the nest and sometimes the mother abandoned them. It was a question of rescuing, fostering and then arranging release for them at a safe and more suitable location. The amazing thing, as far as I was concerned, was that the ducks return year after year to the same sites for breeding – they don't seem to learn from their mistakes!

The court case took all day and was scrupulously fair. Every shred of evidence was taken into account, every angle considered, and every witness cross-examined. I was subjected to a thorough questioning by the defending barrister. I spent almost an hour in the witness box, and remained in court for the remainder of the hearing to advise the prosecuting barrister. An hour later the judge and magistrates retired to consider their decision. When they returned, they dismissed the appeal and upheld the original disqualification. This marked for us the end of a long day and a protracted case. At last the dogs could be rehomed. I drove to my own home a happy man and was surprised at how shattered I felt. It had been a day of immense concentration, and I was asleep by nine thirty that evening.

The next day, after nearly ten hours sleep, I was ready for work, feeling refreshed – which was just as well since we were in for a busy one and on top of that I had a night duty to follow. Normally the onset of warm weather around this time of the year coincides with an upturn in our workload. Although the outpatient numbers hadn't increased yet, there had been an alarming growth in the operating list over the last twenty-four hours. Last night Jeremy had had a quiet time until midnight but then three emergencies had come in in two hours. Two of these were road traffic accidents – one a cat, the other a dog, both with broken thigh bones that would need an X-ray. They had received standard treatment for shock, with a drip and painkillers, and surgery would be done in the morning, if the animals were stabilized and judged fit enough. The other case was a gastric torsion, an extreme emergency that always seems to occur at the dead of night. In this condition, the stomach twists on itself and becomes sealed so that gas accumulating within it cannot be passed out or further down the intestines. The result is a dramatic increase of gas in the stomach, which consequently bloats out. It nearly always occurs in big-chested large dogs, and Jeremy's case was a big fat German shepherd. Night duty is part of veterinary practice and no one begrudges the true emergency and they don't come more urgent than gastric torsions. These emergencies have always been stressful for me, particularly as my first three cases were all fatal in spite of the help of an experienced boss. Getting up at two or three in the morning with the prospect of an hour or two of operating with a high mortality rate is another factor which doesn't delight most veterinary surgeons either. Jeremy had been there within minutes to find the poor dog in a dreadful state. His owner had been woken up by the dog trying to vomit and crying out. At twelve, he was old for a German shepherd but, apart from being fat, had been perfectly healthy all his life. Now, though, the tremendous swelling of Basil's stomach was obvious to anyone: you could tap the side and it was as tight as a drum. He was in agony and would die unless something was done quickly.

There are various techniques for treatment but the most important thing is to get the gas out, relieve pain, treat shock, and then sort out the twisted stomach. Sometimes it is best done all at once but Jeremy's case was too advanced for that. He injected local anaesthetic in a ring round the skin overlying the most distended part of the stomach. He then made an incision to expose the stomach wall and carefully stitched the wall to the skin. Then the most important bit, which would hopefully save Basil's life. Standing well

61

back and using a scalpel he made a large hole in the stomach wall. With a tremendous whoosh the trapped gas burst out, filling the prep room with its smell. Meanwhile, a drip was set up and powerful painkillers given into the vein. The plan was to stabilize Basil so that he presented much less of an anaesthetic risk when the final part of his treatment was undertaken: the untwisting of the stomach.

By the morning all three emergency cases were stable and ready for surgery. Helen performed Basil's operation, which went to plan, and Gabriel mended one of the fractures while I did the other. During the morning two womb infections came in, which needed emergency hysterectomies, and a cat with a blocked bladder – all this in addition to the four major operations already booked in and twenty or so minors. By six the list was just about finished and the hospital fell quiet for a few hours. After a hurried dinner I was back in by seven-thirty for the beginning of my night duty.

The first part of this is always a tour round the hospital to check the in-patients. On the board outside the prep room, the theatre supervisor will have left a list of those patients which need checking following surgery. These would mainly be the difficult or life-threatening cases, and Basil of course was on the list. Usually there are at least six animals to check and I like to do these first. I was halfway through examining Basil, who was doing quite well considering what he had been through, when I was called by Sue, one of the night nurses. A rude, aggressive man was in the waiting room with his dog, which had been limping slightly for a week: he wanted it seen *now*. Sue had checked the dog, found nothing wrong and advised the owner to come back in the morning, as it wasn't an emergency. At this Mr Dodd, the owner, became almost incandescent with rage.

'Tell him he will be seen in half an hour when I've finished my rounds,' I told Sue.

Mr Dodd accepted this with bad grace but settled down in the waiting room. Fortunately he was the only person there.

Halfway through my mini ward rounds, I checked Tiger, the blocked-bladder cat, who now had a catheter. Somehow he had managed to pull it out and his bladder had blocked again. It was rock hard – just like a cricket ball. Sue's colleague, Jackie, and I took Tiger back into the prep room and he had his second anaesthetic of the day while I struggled to put in a new catheter. This involves threading the catheter up the urethra, the tube which goes from the bladder to the outside. Suddenly it went in nicely – most probably I had flushed the obstruction of fine gravel material back into the bladder.

I had forgotten all about Mr Dodd. He was now swearing and shouting and threatening to 'write to the newspapers' to tell them what really went on at the Animal Hospital.

I popped my head round the corner of the waiting room and said, 'You'll be seen in a couple of minutes. Please be patient! The nurse has told you what I've been doing. I'm sure you wouldn't like to be kept waiting if you had a blocked bladder!' This didn't seem to mollify him but at least he stopped pestering the nurse as to how long I was going to be. His dog had sat patiently all the while, much better behaved than his owner.

Just as I was about to see Mr Dodd a police car arrived. This nearly always means bad news and, sure enough, a burly policeman appeared at the door with a badly injured little mongrel in his arms. The semi-conscious dog had been kicked in the face, which was covered with blood, by a man who had been fighting with his owner. All thoughts of Mr Dodd and his limping dog went out of my mind.

Fortunately the presence of the two policemen had a strangely calming effect on him and he sat down quietly while we admitted the latest emergency. Apparently the police had been called to a disturbance between the two men, neighbours, who had been drinking together and had fallen out. One man had been seen to kick the dog, well known and a favourite on the estate, and as soon as the police arrived he was taken into custody – 'for his own safety', as one of the officers put it. We sedated the dog, put him on a drip and cleaned up his wounds. The blood was coming from his nose and ears and one of his eyes was badly bruised. The whereabouts of the owner wasn't known. We invited the police to have a cup of tea, which I needed too by this time. Mr Dodd could wait another ten minutes.

My tea-break lasted only five minutes because Kieran, the ambulance driver, came rushing round to the back with a cat screaming in pain. He had gone out to help an old woman, an invalid, whose cat was her only companion. Whisky had come home bleeding from a leg wound and in distress. During the journey to the hospital, he had got a lot worse. He was now in such agony that I gave an anaesthetic straight away so that I could see what the wound was and why it was causing so much pain. Five minutes later I had more than an inkling as to what it might be. Once cleaned up, the wound was round and neat. It looked as if an air-gun pellet had caused it, which an X-ray confirmed. It had lodged inside the stifle (knee) joint and would have to come out right away. It would be a relatively simple operation and once the pellet was out the pain would be manageable. The police were keen to see this – and as the shooting of the cat had occurred on their patch they told Kieran that they would make enquiries. If nothing else it might scare the delinquent who had shot the cat into not doing it again.

In the event I was grateful for the police presence because Sue came to me again and said that a man was yelling outside the door demanding to be let in. Furthermore he seemed to be drunk. When we opened the door it turned out to be the kicked dog's owner. He still seemed to be fighting mad, with intermittent crying over his dog. I tried to explain that the dog was semi-conscious, but this only provoked him into beating his head against the wall. The policemen intervened and, with great courtesy, suggested that he go home to sober up and see how things were in the morning. This only brought forth a torrent of abuse and, after one firm warning, he was promptly arrested and carted off to the station to spend the night in the cells.

When the police left, it seemed very quiet and I turned to Mr Dodd. It was now half past ten and he had been waiting four hours. But it was a chastened individual who now confronted me. 'I'm sorry to trouble you, mate,' he said. 'I didn't realize you were so busy!' I think somehow he had quite enjoyed the dramas that had unfolded over the evening. Maybe he had got the message about what constitutes an emergency. His dog had some pain at the back of the leg and I thought it probably wasn't anything worse than a pulled muscle. I had had plenty of experience of those myself when I was an athlete at university. Rest and some anti-inflammatory pills should sort it out within three weeks, I said.

Back in the wards Whisky had come round and was purring. A very nice contrast. Basil, the gastric-torsion dog, was making progress and looked as though he would pull through, and the dog with facial injuries was comfortable but still not properly conscious. The nurse would tend him overnight. It was time for me to get some rest.

Boring it isn't, I thought, as I pulled into the drive at home.

Next day, checking my patients of the night before, I was glad to see that twelve hours' rest and pain-relief had improved the terrier. He was now able to stand although his head was still painful to the touch. Another two days in hospital should see him right, I thought, and then he could go home. A visit from one of our inspectors would also make sure that he was being looked after properly.

I needed, and got, a quiet day after all the excitement of the previous twenty-four hours, and by five o'clock I was ready for an evening at home with the family.

MAY

At last the weather really warmed up. When I look back to my distant college days, I think of May and tennis after lectures, particularly in the final year when we all lived in the country, and also the start of the athletics season with (mostly) warm summer evenings. It wasn't too long before some lovely weather brightened the whole hospital as the work increased. Fleas are one reason for this, but also people are out and about more with their dogs, which offers more opportunities for mishaps. But one of the first cases of the month was something quite unusual.

At ten Bibi was not old for a miniature poodle: this breed often gets to fourteen or fifteen before succumbing to serious illness. In fact, a month ago her mother had been put down when we discovered she had breast cancer, which had spread to the lungs. Ever since then Bibi had gone off her food and her owner, Mary, who had been widowed only six months earlier, had at first thought that the dog was pining for her mother. They had had a close bond and Bibi was still looking for her every day. When Bibi continued to refuse to eat, Mary became really worried and brought her in for examination.

Over the following week several of the vets saw her but no physical explanation could be found for her lack of appetite. Mary was becoming frantic – Bibi was getting thinner by the day and looked unhappy. Eventually, after three weeks of not eating, Stan admitted her for blood and urine tests and observation.

The routine blood tests for sick animals consist of a screen of the red and white blood cells and 'serum biochemistry', which measures various enzymes, proteins and waste products, which gives us information about the liver and kidneys in particular. A day later all the results came back normal. I had looked at the blood screen for evidence of infection – this would show by an increase in the white blood cells – but everything was in the normal range. Overnight, Trudy, one of the night nurses, had managed to get some chicken into Bibi but only by petting her and hand feeding her bit by bit. It was looking increasingly as if Mary's original diagnosis, pining, was the right one. As the hospital was filling up, we had to send Bibi home and could only suggest to Mary that she persevere with tender loving care and patience.

A week later Mary was back. Bibi was still only picking at her food. It seemed that the only thing we hadn't tried was a companion for her and Mary had come to the same conclusion. She set off round the RSPCA homing centres and, just by chance, a small female crossbred dog of nine years old had been handed in: the owner had had to move into sheltered accommodation. But would the two dogs get on? I thought Mary should try for three weeks and wait and see.

Meanwhile, my thoughts were on a different problem, but in another miniature poodle. Unlike Bibi, Suki's problem was a voracious appetite, incessant thirst, wetting indoors, and an alarming loss of weight. She was ten too, and had just finished her season. It had been going on for a week or so, but when Joan and Roy, her owners, thought about it, the drinking had been increasing gradually for a couple of months. The wetting in the house had been attributed at first to increasing age, and allowance made, but over the last week it was obvious that something was seriously wrong. The house was beginning to smell too in spite of intensive cleaning sessions.

With symptoms like this my thoughts went straight to diabetes mellitus – or sugar diabetes. This is quite common in dogs and it's a little known fact that the discoverers of the disease, Drs Banting and Best, had studied the disease in them. Of course, there are many other reasons for a dog to drink excessively and be unable to control its bladder but a urine test would set the ball rolling towards an accurate diagnosis. Roy and Joan were handed a small tray and a pot and sent outside with instructions to catch a little in the tray when Suki squatted, then transfer it to the pot. They were a cheerful couple in their fifties, whom we had seen a few times in the hospital with their pet. Roy had been made redundant three times and this time was finding it much more difficult to return to work. In spite of this the pair of them managed to have a laugh when they came in and didn't seem to mind the odd looks outside the hospital as they followed Suki about with a small stainless steel tray. A few minutes later, Roy came back, happily displaying a half-full pot to the nearly full waiting room. There were a few chuckles and questions as to where he had got it from, did he realize this was an animal hospital and comments along those lines before I got to checking out the sample.

One minute later I was fairly certain that Suki had diabetes: the paper strip I had dipped into the urine had gone bright green, indicating the presence of glucose.

Since I qualified there have been phenomenal developments in the diagnosis and treatment of this condition in dogs. Nowadays diabetic dogs are frequently kept in hospital while the correct dose of insulin is worked out. This can be done with serial blood-glucose estimations made over a twenty-four-hour period and recorded on a graph. It's an area of veterinary medicine that Gabriel loves and he is often to be seen poring over the results of the blood-glucose measurements. But before I admitted Suki there would be one thing to get straight with the owners: their willingness and ability to cope with the treatment. Nothing short of total commitment will do. They would have to be taught a great deal: how to test urine, give insulin injections and recognize the signs of overdose, for example. Injections would be necessary every day for the rest of the dog's life, which could be another four years or so, and they would, of course, have to make arrangements for her during holidays.

I had every confidence in Roy and Joan, but you never can tell until you start the teaching process and go through the first few months. Some owners give up easily while others do well but can't manage if problems arise. Others surprise you by being brilliant at the whole thing when you didn't expect it.

I remember particularly an old lady who found it difficult to understand anything I said to her about the disease. She failed to inject the dog the first half-dozen times and found everything too complicated. I quickly realized that the problem was her lack of confidence in her ability to get to grips with anything complicated, especially when it was me doing the explaining! I did what I have found to be best ever since and left her with the nurse to go through everything bit by bit. Janine, who had immense patience, took over the day-to-day management of the case, with me checking every week. Once the old lady got the hang of it all she managed splendidly. Over the next four years she kept her dog beautifully stabilized, only rarely needing to do urine checks. She was able to adjust the insulin dose based on the dog's appetite, thirst and general alertness. In four years we had no problems and the dog eventually died of something not connected with the diabetes. In all my years as a vet I haven't seen a more astute owner in dealing with the disease.

As I had expected, Roy and Joan were keen to take on Suki's treatment and I explained what would happen next. Gabriel, with his fascination for diabetes, almost inevitably ended up with the day-to-day stabilization of the dog. Lots of blood samples were taken, graphs plotted and insulin doses calculated. Typically, a dog will spend at least five days in the hospital while the correct dose of insulin is established. Meanwhile, the nurses spend half an hour each morning educating the owners in how to inject their dog, test urine and what to look for if too much insulin is given and the blood glucose goes too low. While the owners are at the hospital they often visit their pet and give the injection, which happens first thing in the morning.

By the end of the week Suki was ready to go home. She was putting on weight, and eating and drinking normally. Roy and Joan were really pleased to have her back, albeit a bit nervous at having to do it all on their own. The first weekend passed uneventfully and they were surprised how easy it all was. I caught up with them in the car park a few days after their first check-up and they told me how much more pleasant it was at home now that they weren't having to clean up after her all the time.

Pets with illnesses that cause mess can put a huge strain on the whole family: not only is there the worry about the illness and its consequences, but there is often considerable guilt if they cannot cope with the mess. Dorothy was at the next consulting session with her old mongrel, Fred. She must have been at least eighty and suffered from arthritis, as did her dog. They both struggled in, Dorothy with her walking stick and Fred with the typical swaying gait of the arthritic dog. They were obviously devoted to each other: Dorothy constantly stroked Fred's head while she told me the history, and he kept looking up at her with adoring eyes, sparing the occasional nervous glance for me. It was as if he had got the drift of the conversation

With great sadness, Dorothy had come to the conclusion that she might have to have him put down. Over the last six months Fred had been a regular visitor to the hospital for his arthritis. It had been kept under reasonable control with drugs but over the last week he had developed diarrhoea, which had not responded to changing his diet to fish and rice. Now he was straining to pass a motion and was passing blood at the same time. Dorothy stood before me with tears in her eyes. It was obvious that she fully expected me to agree that Fred should be put to sleep. After all, he was sixteen. However, I always think it is best just to check the animal over to be sure that the owner is making the right decision – particularly when they are as upset as Dorothy was. The thing that struck me about Fred was that for such an old dog he was bright and alert. Apart from his stiff hindquarters, he didn't look like a dog that had come to the end of his days. After going over him I felt that he had all the symptoms of colitis, which is inflammation of the colon and common in dogs (and humans). Straining to pass motions after a period of diarrhoea, then passing blood, are suggestive of the disease.

'How about if I take him in for a few days and see if I can sort him out?' I suggested.

Dorothy looked up, hardly believing her ears. 'Do you think you can?'

'No promises, but if it's colitis he might be better in a few days and we can try different arthritis pills, too, as they may be helping to cause the problem. At any rate, there's no harm in trying.' It was almost as if Dorothy herself had had a reprieve from the grim consequences of serious illness: her tears were replaced by a hopeful smile.

Fred duly trotted after Lisa, the nurse who was to admit him. He even managed to look less stiff than when he had come in, perhaps thinking he was going home. The difference between a dog's demeanour before and after a consultation is always striking: many leap for joy as soon as they are off the table, having had to be dragged into the room.

In the afternoon I had another look at Fred because I had to decide whether to treat him for colitis without extensive tests including X-rays. I decided to put him on treatment for a few days: at his age I didn't want to get into general anaesthetics. I checked first for any obvious growths and also his prostate gland, enlargement of which is a common problem in old dogs and something we see virtually every week. The treatment for this is castration, which may sound a bit drastic but is highly effective. By coincidence, Bairbre was in the middle of castrating a dog in the adjacent operating theatre for this reason. Fred's prostate was normal, though. He was given an injection of antibiotic and steroid and put on a special drug for colitis. At the end of the working day I glanced at him in his cage and was pleased to see him tucking into some chicken, which the nurses had cooked for him. No sign of separation anxiety there in spite of his many years.

In fact separation anxiety was my first case of the next afternoon – quite a common complaint which is, nevertheless, potentially time-consuming. Ron and Maria Jones had acquired their dog six months ago from a rescue agency. He was a six-month-old mongrel, who had been thrown out of a car, which then sped off. They called him Lucky and almost immediately he had settled into a loving home as if he had always lived there. The couple were pensioners and so were able to be with him all the time during the settling-in period. The problems began whenever they went out together: Lucky just couldn't bear to be left alone. Curiously he would retreat to the toilet, open the door and stay there pawing at the door and barking constantly until his owner returned.

A lot of dogs with separation anxiety are destructive and the condition has well-known patterns. The anxious behaviour begins almost immediately the owners leave and consists of chewing, soiling, scratching and incessant howling – Lucky's speciality, which led to the inevitable complaint from neighbours who were otherwise good friends of Ron and Maria. Why Lucky chose to do it in the toilet remained a mystery!

The fact that the undesirable behaviour begins almost immediately the owners leave has led to a programme that tries to break the pattern. Trigger factors tend to set off these dogs. They learn quickly to recognize the signs that the owners are going out – for example, picking up keys, turning off the television, putting on a coat – and get worked up if it looks as though they aren't going to be included in the outing. It has also been found that most really destructive behaviour occurs in the first few minutes that the dog is alone.

A typical initial programme to try to reverse the undesirable behaviour patterns might be not to turn off the television, and not to make a ritual of leaving. We advise owners to leave quietly, return within thirty seconds and pet the dog if he hasn't started trashing the place or howling. Over a short time, the owners are asked to leave many times, always coming back quickly, at varying times in the first phase, then gradually lengthening the time before returning, so that at the end of the day the dog is used to the idea that the owners always come back, and often sooner rather than later. In many cases, depending on the owners' persistence and patience, separation anxiety can be resolved – within a matter of weeks in the best cases.

In the time that I had available, which was less than ideal, I put these ideas to Ron and his wife. Fortunately, they had the time, and probably the patience, to give it a go. Maria was quite amused because her granddaughter of two and a half was playing up at night, refusing to go to bed or waking up crying and wanting stories. Her mother was in the middle of a programme not dissimilar from Lucky's.

'What happens if this doesn't work?' said Ron, always the worrier of the two. 'Could he not just be given tranquillizers whenever we go out?'

'I don't like giving dogs sedatives in the long term,' I said. 'They never sort out the basic problem and may not work anyway. Maybe for Bonfire Night they're OK but otherwise it's not a good idea.'

The couple left with a time limit of three weeks to see if the basic plan would make an improvement. I reckoned Maria would be the driving force – and I looked forward to hearing how her granddaughter was getting on too, having been in the same situation myself with my elder daughter!

As I have said many times, one of the joys of being a veterinary surgeon is the sheer variety of the work, even in an inner-city veterinary hospital – my country colleagues in mixed practice have even more choice of patients and conditions to learn about. The next day we were confronted with something for which we lack expertise and the facilities to deal with; we could offer only short-term first aid.

RSPCA Inspector John Bowe and his colleagues had

been called to a large number of oiled ducks on a river to the north of London. They weren't sure how the oil had been spilled but the effect on the ducks was dramatic – they were covered in it. Many were transported to the RSPCA wildlife hospital in Norfolk but half a dozen were too ill to be taken there immediately and were brought to the Harmsworth. I had telephoned the Norfolk hospital for advice and, as always, they had been very helpful. The worst of the oil was cleaned off and the ducks were stomach-tubed and given rehydrating fluids, containing salts and glucose. They were then bedded down on thick towels. Having been to a lecture on oiled birds, I recognized that we couldn't treat them fully at the Harmsworth: the washing process uses water under quite considerable pressure and is lengthy. Also lengthy is the recuperation period during which the natural oils that make ducks buoyant return to the feathers. It might be weeks before they could be released into the wild. As I watched them being loaded into the van for Norfolk, I thought they seemed a bit better than they had when they arrived, but only time would tell.

Meanwhile, on ward rounds, I found that Fred was doing well. He had had two days on a drug called salazopyrin for his colitis, was much brighter and had passed no more blood. Jala, the reports nurse, phoned Dorothy to see if she would like to try the dog at home. No problem there! She was delighted to hear that Fred was rallying – and I was pleased not only for the dog but also to have another free cage. Just like the NHS, we are under constant pressure for 'beds'. Fred had responded well and I had high hopes for a complete cure, at least in the short term, although colitis tends to recur. It might be that we would have to manage relapses as and when they happened but we could cross that bridge when we came to it.

The hospital was bulging at the seams and it was not even summer yet. Looking down the operations list I was relieved to see that most of the major operations were relatively straightforward and that the patients should not need to stay in, especially if we could do them in the morning session. My first op was on an old female crossbreed dog with cancer of the breast. This is a common disease so that not a day goes past without a case. My patient was called Bessy and it was the first time I had seen her. One disadvantage of working in a big animal hospital is that you don't necessarily have the close contact with the owner that you would in a smaller set-up. Bessy had been seen with an infected mammary growth by Jeremy, who had prescribed antibiotics. Stan had checked her out a week later and prescribed a further course of antibiotics to clear up the remaining infection. Helen had done the next check and booked a pre-operation X-ray to make sure that the cancer had not spread to the lungs, and a blood test to establish that the liver and kidneys were functioning well and that the infection was under control. There was a note on the card saying that Bessy's owner was desperately worried and we were to phone immediately if there were any problems.

The operation consists of removing the mammary gland containing the cancer. It's called a radical mastectomy and it must be thorough, or there is a big risk that the cancer will return. It is not a difficult operation to perform but is time-consuming. Much of the hour-and-a-half was taken up with putting in lots and lots of stitches. In spite of being thirteen, Bessy was quickly round from the anaesthetic and would go home the same day. We had recently switched to a new gas anaesthetic and recovery times were amazingly quick – sometimes, as in Bessy's case, within minutes of finishing the operation. The final chore was to write up the clinical notes so that the next vet would know exactly what had been done. While I was doing this it occurred to me that I had never met Bessy's owner, and I would probably not see the results of my labours: almost inevitably I would be somewhere else when the stitches came out. If Bessy made a complete recovery, today would be the last time I would see her, likely as not. Chatting to owners before the operation, reassuring them afterwards and seeing the successful results of your labours are some of the pleasures of the job I tend to miss out on.

Andrew, the nurse who assisted during the operation, took Bessy back into her ward, then returned to package the cancerous tissue and send it off for analysis. I had reasonable hopes that it would be benign, in which case we would consider Bessy cured.

It wasn't just the caseload that was increasing. In my office I can see from a glance at my phone how many incoming calls we are receiving. In the last week or so there had been a huge number and, as each call is logged, I flicked through the phone book to see why. About 20 per cent had been to do with fledglings. My heart sank. In spite of innumerable messages from the RSPCA and the Royal Society for the Protection of Birds (RSPB), every year a large number of young birds that have just left the nest are brought into the hospital as having been 'abandoned'. The simple message in the RSPCA leaflet says, 'Don't touch! If you find a baby bird please leave it alone! The parent birds are probably collecting food, or waiting nearby – they won't come back until you've gone.' It goes on to say that if the fledgling is on a road it can be moved to a safer spot nearby; if you are worried, leave the bird for an hour or so and then return. In most instances, the parents will have taken care of their youngster. Even though the advice is the best available, and agreed by two major charities with expertise in the area, it often falls on deaf ears and, at worst, leads to verbal abuse on the phone.

When fledglings turn up at the hospital doors, having been brought sometimes quite long distances by well-meaning but misguided people, we have no alternative but to take them in, which quickly fills up ward eight. The nurses do their best, and we try to shift as many as possible to wildlife centres but many, sadly, don't survive. They would have had a much better chance if left alone. Even if they survive and learn to fly, we do not know how they will adapt once released. The parents are so important to them in those first few weeks.

The next day in ward eight we had half a dozen fledglings, mainly blackbirds but also a magpie, the inevitable ducklings and a gosling. Bairbre had removed a bit of discarded fishing line from the gosling's mouth the night before and we had to find somewhere for it to go. Thank goodness for the swan sanctuary, I thought. They take all sorts for rehabilitation, not just swans and, hopefully, they would be able to help. Clare was feeding the fledglings, whose gaping beaks were appealing, but it would take a determined effort to ensure their survival.

During the morning operations the clouds began to thicken and we heard dramatic crashes of thunder, followed soon by torrential rain. I could hardly see as I set off to drive to an outside clinic. I doubted whether many owners would brave the downpour if it continued and it showed no sign of abating. We have two satellite clinics in north London to relieve the pressure on the hospital outpatients department. We don't do any operating in the clinics and I usually expect to see about thirty animals in each session, but on a day like this I'd be lucky to see ten. As expected, it was a small, bedraggled crowd that greeted me as I arrived. There were no dogs in the waiting room, which didn't surprise me as dogs are often frightened by thunderstorms. There were just two hamsters, four cats and a budgie. The first hamster in was quite straightforward: his front teeth needed clipping.

Then in trudged a worried-looking Judy and her small daughter, Jennifer, with their hamster Perdita. 'She's a year old and Jennifer has seen some lumps on her tummy,' said Judy. 'I'm worried they could be growths.'

Perdita looked in splendid condition but was not in a good mood. Hamsters are nocturnal creatures and can get quite grumpy if woken up suddenly, although I couldn't believe that she had been able to sleep with the storm we were having.

I turned her over carefully. 'Why do you call him Perdita?' I asked.

There was a silence, then Judy replied, 'We were told it was a female by the pet shop.'

A thought occurred to me. 'Are these the lumps you're worried about?' I pointed to the testicles. I think the penny was beginning to drop because a red-faced Judy said nothing and looked at her daughter, who hadn't been following the conversation and was now demanding an explanation as to what was going on. Like all young children, she knew enough about the possible consequences of illness to worry about her pet.

'There's nothing to worry about, Jennifer,' I said. 'Perdita's a boy and you're going to have to change her name! Your mum will explain.' After a few minutes, Judy saw the funny side and laughed. It wasn't long before the pair of them were at it. They decided to sit in the waiting room while the rain was at its worst, and the chuckles coming from there told me that they hadn't kept secret the news of Perdita's sex change.

The cats were simple cases – flu, flea allergies and a case of cystitis (inflammation of the bladder) that was causing the poor cat constantly to visit the litter tray. It had been going on since last night and the owner had seen some blood in the urine. Most such cases respond to antibiotics although if it keeps coming back a special diet may be required to change the acidity of the urine The budgie was simpler still, only needing its beak and claws trimmed. No more patients turned up and I spent half an hour nattering to the manager of the clinic, Terry, whom I have known for twenty-five years. Between us we know hundreds of people who have worked at the Harmsworth and Terry has kept in contact with many of them. Some of the stories he comes up with have me in fits of laughter. Certainly the Harmsworth was and still is a fund of anecdotes, some of which defy belief.

With the rain abating, I drove straight home, arriving earlier than usual and with a couple of days off to look forward to. The weather had made for a quiet, stress-free day, which was a nice change from the usual buzz. When it has been quiet, it is easier to switch off and get into family things. Learning to relax more effectively was one of my New Year resolutions and I'm still working on it!

JUNE

The beginning of the summer brought an acute shortage of space. Ward seven was again full of stray cats – it's a never-ending problem. For the first time I could remember we found ourselves with more than thirty healthy cats to try to place in homing centres, not to mention a dozen kittens. At this rate, I thought, we'll be cancelling operations unless we can shift some. Andy, the reports nurse for this week, set about the interminable phone calls that might bring relief. And it wasn't just cats that had found their way to us: in ward eight there were two cockerels, a couple of hens, three hamsters, rats, hedgehogs, two cockatiels (we're never without at least one in the exotics ward), a fledgling black-bird, four crows and two magpies. And this was supposed to be inner London! Most of these creatures arrived without a lot wrong with them but feeding and cleaning them out ties up valuable nurses.

Just when I was about to tear my hair out, help was at hand. Our Kent friends came up trumps yet again and found spaces for ten cats. Another ten went to homing centres all over the place. Andrew, one of the ambulance drivers, came to take most of the wildlife to a wildlife centre and suddenly, within a day, the pressure was off – at least for the time being. Even the cockerels were found somewhere to live: on a city farm. We were lucky as they are quite difficult to place. I find them amusing and charming but I don't have to put up with them crowing at the crack of dawn. I often wonder how on earth cockerels come to be wandering up busy high roads in the East End of London, but it isn't uncommon.

They talk about flaming June but it seemed to have done nothing but tank down since the month started. No wonder we stopped hearing about hosepipe bans! Rain kept the clinics quiet, as most people don't venture out in it unless it's absolutely necessary. Ginny, a young guinea-pig, couldn't wait for better weather though – she was in need of urgent attention. Her skin was very itchy and, according to her nine-year-old owner, Samantha, this had crept up on her. The guinea-pig had been scratching for a few weeks and Samantha had noticed a flea on her fur. She had treated this with some flea powder, which she had bought for her cat. Cuddles the cat liked to cuddle up to the guinea-pig and they seemed to be pals, so the flea had explained away the itchiness. But, all of a sudden, it had got really bad, and Ginny had lost most of her hair. Worse, she now had some sores from her constant scratching. She was obviously in some distress: she had gone off her food and become irritable – not wanting anything to do with the cat and crying out in that high-pitched squeak guinea pigs give when they are unhappy.

It was pretty obvious what was wrong with Ginny because she had all the telltale symptoms: guinea-pig mange, caused by a mite called *Tryxacarus caviae*. This mite is usually quite easy to find on skin scrapings so I did one and looked down the microscope a few minutes later. There they were – diagnosis confirmed! – and Samantha wrinkled her nose in disgust when she saw the little mites scurrying about.

If not treated, mange in guinea-pigs can prove fatal, with the animal developing convulsions, so the sooner we got things under control the better. For many years I pre-scribed a medicated shampoo but unfortunately owners didn't always use it properly. It was also messy, had to be repeated every week for up to a month and, most important of all, the guinea-pig hated it. Nowadays, we inject them with a relatively new drug, ivermectin. It is mainly used for the control of parasites in cattle and horses but it has found favour in guinea-pigs too. An injection, repeated in ten days, usually does the trick.

Guinea-pigs are interesting creatures. Their scientific name is *Cavia porcellus*, which gives rise to their other name, cavy. Native to South America, they are popular children's pets but in their original habitat they are not kept as pets at all. Some years ago during travels around Peru, I got into conversation with a Quechua-speaking Indian (for-tunately for me he also spoke some English!) and the topic of guinea-pigs came up. It turned out that they are consid-ered a delicacy, especially for wedding feasts and, accord-ing to my new friend, at wedding anniversaries. 'A wedding anniversary wouldn't be the same without guinea-pig,' he told me solemnly. Samantha would have been horrified if she knew.

Another interesting feature of guinea-pigs is that, like us, they are susceptible to vitamin C deficiency. Of course, in humans vitamin C deficiency is unheard-of on a normal diet. It was, though, a common disease in sailors before the cause and remedy was discovered. In sailors deprived of fresh fruit, high in vitamin C, scurvy resulted: it caused bleeding from the gums and teeth to fall out, among other things.

Guinea-pigs are unable to synthesise vitamin C in their bodies and must, therefore, be given enough in their diet. Mistakes are often made with their food, as is often the case with most exotic pets, and I saw a case of scurvy in a guinea-pig a few days after I had treated Ginny. Piggy was so named because he always seemed hungry. His owners, Ruth and her daughter Rachel, fed him on pellets without any greens: a year or two before, he had had a spell of diarrhoea after eating some lettuce, and the pet shop had told his owners that the pellets contained everything he needed. This is true to an extent, but if the pellets go stale, especially if they are older than three months, then vitamin C levels may drop.

Before going on holiday Ruth had bought twice the normal amount of pellets because the neighbours would be feeding Piggy. When they returned Piggy had been off his food but he picked up as soon as the family were together again. Rachel noticed that the food seemed stale, but Piggy ate it, although more slowly than usual.

A few weeks passed and then, all of a sudden, he went downhill. He seemed unsteady on his legs, had lost quite a bit of weight (it's surprising how easy it is to miss that a pet has lost weight under its fur) and was generally under the weather. A deficiency of vitamin C, either absolute or marginal, is at the back of every vet's mind when looking at sick guinea-pigs and Piggy's diet, especially the lack of greens and possibly stale pellets, made me suspicious.

Nothing else fitted with him, so I prescribed 100 mg of vitamin C daily. This was easily achieved by breaking up a tablet intended for humans and diluting it in his drinking water. Over the next month he would need to be put on a more balanced diet of fresh pellets, greens and good hay. Within days he was picking up and it looked as though we were on the right track. When I looked up scurvy in the guinea-pig books I found that it could cause bleeding in the gums, just as in people, and also bleeding in the joints.

It's quite amazing how commonly an incorrect diet causes disease. With the advent of 'designer' and exotic pets, incorrect feeding figures high in diagnosis of illness. I wonder just how careful some pet shops are in ensuring that a new owner is given enough information on the care of a new pet. Piggy, though, had been unlucky, with a combination of unusual circumstances leading to his vitamin deficiency.

I can never understand what drives people to keep some of the animals we see. Dogs and cats are so loving and well adapted to people, so many need good, caring homes, why go for the exotic and bizarre? And talking of truly bizarre we were in for a real surprise in the middle of the month. I thought I had seen everything in inner-London veterinary practice but I was wrong. A man was exercising his friend's dog in a south London park when the dog began to play with something in the long grass. Curious, he went over to have a look and saw what he took to be a lizard. He picked it up – a mistake, because he received a nasty bite, which made him drop it. Not daunted, he found a blanket, put it over the animal and took it home. This Good Samaritan caringly put the lizard in his pond overnight – his second mistake, because it ate the three terrapins that were living there. Then he called the RSPCA.

Inspector Megan Jones was amazed to see that the 'lizard' was a crocodile. Not a big one, admittedly – it was only sixteen inches long – but big enough to be dangerous. With the help of the RSPCA, it was transported to London Zoo where the reptile experts identified it as *Caiman crocodilus*, or the spectacled caiman. This is native to Central America so it is interesting to speculate on what it was doing in a south London park. The zoo was unable to accept it as they have a strict policy on introducing new stock to their collection in order to prevent disease. The crocodile was brought to the hospital while we sorted out somewhere for it to go. In its special glass cage, it proved something of a curiosity for the staff.

Talking to one of our group inspectors, Mark Martin, I was astonished to find out that it was easy to buy crocodiles in London. And poisonous spiders, snakes, tarantulas and even a deadly species of octopus too. Although a licence to keep dangerous animals is a requirement in law, this is in most cases a mere formality and not necessarily pointed out to potential owners. I was told that the crocodile had been bought probably on a whim for a hundred pounds or less, and would almost certainly have been abandoned when the owner found out how difficult such animals are to keep properly. Another factor might have been the knowledge that, when fully grown, caimans may reach up to eight feet in length. By which time it would be truly dangerous.

We are fortunate to have the help of the British Reptile and Amphibian Society who regularly bail us out whenever – increasingly frequently – we are landed with exotic reptiles. They came to our aid within twenty-four hours in the form of Mick Powell, a hard-working Society member, who moved the caiman to an expert with the knowledge and facilities to look after it properly. Before it went I had a look at it in its temporary accommodation. It hardly moved, but its unblinking stare was sufficient to raise the hairs on the back of my neck. Perhaps it's a disturbing sign of the times, but in other parts of the country similarly dangerous animals have turned up. It worries me because at the hospital we are so often in the front line to deal with these creatures when they are abandoned.

Thankfully, that evening on night duty, it was back to the more mundane things with which I am familiar. In the space of one hour I had a West Highland white terrier which had collided with a bus, a sixteen-year-old golden retriever with an infected womb, and a cat with a suspected foreign body in her throat She was gagging, and had been for four days!

First the accident. Considering that the Westie had chosen a bus with which to get involved, he was in surprisingly good shape. The main worry with all accidents is shock, which is the first thing to check for in the initial assessment. An animal is in shock when the blood pressure drops – for example, after an accident which causes loss of blood. The maintenance of an adequate blood supply to the vital organs, such as the brain, is endangered and if untreated may lead to a downward spiral and death. Judging by his rather pale colour, Jamie was shocked. The easiest way to check a dog's colour is by looking inside the cheek at the mucous membranes. They should be a nice red colour but in Jamie's case they were pale pink. The other useful test is to push your thumb against the mucous membrane so that it goes white and then watch how quickly the colour returns – it should be almost instantaneous. With shocked animals, it may take two or three seconds. This test is called the capillary refill time, and is a rough measure of whether the blood is circulating properly. In addition to being pale, Jamie had a sluggish capillary refill, indicating that he needed treatment for shock, which was only to be expected. Apart from shock I couldn't find any injuries so, although shock alone can kill, I was hopeful that he would make it. This information was conveyed to his anxious owners who were waiting at home for news.

Their story was not typical. Most of the road traffic accidents that I have seen over the years have been caused by dogs not on a lead. It only needs something tempting, like another dog or even better a cat, for a dog to run into the road. Poor Jamie had been on a flexi-lead that had not locked. He had simply meandered into the path of the bus, which was gliding silently along beside the pavement, was bowled over and landed in a heap in the gutter. Fortunately, a police car was passing by and the officers brought him into the hospital wrapped in a blanket. The nurses put him on a drip as soon as I had finished looking at him. The fluids passing into his circulation would bring his pressure up and get him stabilized.

Meanwhile, my attention turned to the old dog with the infected womb. The only treatment for this would be a hysterectomy, but before surgery she, too, would need a drip. However, there was a problem: because of her age there was great uncertainty whether to operate or put her to sleep. Two of the family who owned her agonized for twenty minutes, then announced that they would have to discuss it with their mum. My advice was to go ahead with the operation – it was the dog's only chance. I couldn't guarantee survival and, of course, it would be impossible to predict how long Shelly would live afterwards. I resolved the matter by setting up the drip and saying that we would operate first thing in the morning, if the family agreed.

Finally, the cat with the possible throat problem. She, too, was old – seventeen – and had been gagging for four days, during which time she had not eaten anything. Her owners, a middle-aged couple, had decided to bring her in, suspecting that she had something stuck in her throat. This always worries me because more often than not nothing is stuck and the animal has an infection at the back of the throat. Every so often, though, the owner is right and the secret is to know when that is! I tried to look but Pippy wasn't having any of it. Like many old cats, she would not

90

brook too much handling, and used her front claws to get at me – even with Emma, the duty nurse, hanging on to her paws. Emma had done a quick check when the cat arrived and thought she had caught a glimpse of something at the back of the throat. Taking her at her word, I decided that the only thing I could do would be to give a quick anaesthetic and have a proper look. Pippy's owners had borrowed a friend's car to get to the hospital and I suggested they stay to find out one way or the other and maybe take their pet home afterwards. I had an eye on the cage situation – there weren't many empty ones and tomorrow there would be more admissions.

A few minutes later I was astonished to see not one but three neat little fish bones stuck firmly at the back of Pippy's throat. Emma and the owners had been right! They were small and had sharp little points at the side, which had been firmly stuck into the throat tissue. I had to use forceps to manipulate them out. It took only a few minutes, and by the time we had drawn up the antibiotic injection and given it, Pippy was stirring.

Her owners were amazed to see the bones and felt guilty to think that they had been there for four days. Neither of them ate fish and they could only surmise that the bones had been the result of a forage into the neighbours' dustbins. Despite her age Pippy had a healthy appetite and enjoyed spending most of her time in the garden, especially at this time of year. Half an hour later she was on her way home, still sleepy but no longer gagging – and very hungry judging by the loud meowing she had started as soon as she came to.

Before setting off for home I checked Jamie. It's truly surprising how resilient animals are. His whole demeanour and colour had taken a turn for the better. There can't be many dogs who survive an altercation with a bus. The next morning you wouldn't have thought that anything had happened at all. There he was, wagging his tail – Westies are usually sociable dogs and Jamie was no exception. The only hint of a problem was when I tried to touch the side of his face. This made him flinch but even then he didn't growl or have a go at me. Just a bit of bruising, and he could go home to his much-relieved owners.

After ward rounds I found myself operating on a dog whose problem made him *too* sociable, at least in the eyes of other male dogs. Benito, a ten-year-old Cavalier King Charles spaniel owned by an Italian family, had started to behave oddly and lose his hair. Mr Vincenzo, his owner who took him for most of his walks, had noticed the baldness first and at first he hadn't been worried. This was unusual because hair loss generally has pet owners hotfooting it to the vet. Perhaps it was that Mr Vincenzo had also lost a generous quantity of hair – which he was proud of, as it happens!

Benito's hair had started to come out on his tummy, then on his flanks and legs. A trip to the vet had been planned but not considered urgent until several other strange things happened. First poor Benito's breasts began to enlarge, as if he were pregnant, and then he stopped cocking his leg when he wanted to urinate, preferring instead to squat like a bitch. Finally, and this was the most disturbing bit, he became an object of desire among the neighbouring male dog population. Even a castrated animal tried to jump upon him after a chance meeting in the park. Worst of all, a particularly persistent beast took to hanging around the house howling intermittently outside the front door. Clearly something was wrong with Benito's hormones and urgent action was required, for everyone's sake.

Benito's story is so typical and his appearance so characteristic of a particular disease that a likely cause of his problem immediately sprang to mind. The likely diagnosis was cancer of the testicle, leading to the production of too much of the female sex hormone, oestrogen. A Sertoli's cell tumour produces this effect and the cancer is seventeen more times likely to occur in an undescended testicle. Many are still in the abdomen and an X-ray may be needed to confirm their presence, while others are partially descended and can be found in the groin, which is much easier to diagnose: the testicle is invariably enlarged, while the normal one, labouring under the influence of the oestrogen, is shrunken. This was exactly the state of affairs with Benito. Mr Vincenzo was astounded that he hadn't noticed the quite large bulge in the dog's groin.

Now came the difficult bit. Mr Vincenzo didn't like the sound of castration but accepted reluctantly that if he wanted some peace and quiet, and also to cure his pet, then the affected testicle, preferably both, would have to come out. It often seems to be our Latin friends who hate the idea of depriving their pet of something they are not even getting! I have had innumerable discussions with various people and some simply refuse to countenance any surgery. In the case of cats they come in time after time with bite wounds from scrapping, and even pointing out that castrated cats live almost twice as long on average doesn't make any difference. But common sense prevailed in Mr Vincenzo's case and I assured his owner that Benito would benefit from having both testicles removed. There would be no possibility that way of any further development of cancer. Sertoli's cell tumour has a low rate of spread so the chances of a total cure were good. And I expected Benito's hair to be growing back like spring grass within three months.

Just before operating we took the precaution of X-raying the dog's chest and abdomen, but as I had hoped and expected there was no sign of spread. Because the cancerous testicle wasn't in the abdomen, the surgery was easy and a quarter of an hour later Benito was having the last stitch put in. He could go home almost straight away. A large extended family was waiting anxiously at home for him – Gran, Granddad, the Vincenzos and their four young children, a cat and, of course, Benito's suitor, who was still hanging around hopefully and bounding up every time the door opened.

Meanwhile, Shelly's family had decided to go ahead with the hysterectomy and Stan had done this while I was operating on Benito. He told me that the op had gone well and that Shelly was sitting up in her cage. Stan also said that he was confident of a full recovery. It looked like the family chat had come up with the best solution.

A few days later I had one of those nice afternoon clinics when all the animals have curable illnesses that are easy to diagnose. Even better, I had several owners in for repeat examinations of their pets and all were doing well. Roy and Joan came first with Suki. What a difference a month had made! She was bright-eyed, had put on weight and bounded into the surgery, wagging her tail and jumping up at me. Her insulin dose had stayed at twenty units daily and this was being given at nine in the morning. Joan had learned to give a third of the dog's food at the same time (so that Suki would know that the injection was always followed by something pleasant) and the remainder was given at four in the afternoon when the insulin level was at its highest. This way, there would be less risk of the glucose level in the blood going too low and causing a coma. Things were going well and the couple had their dog back as a normal healthy

94

pet. The routine was simple and they were doing spot checks on the urine from time to time.

Next in were Ron and Maria with Lucky. They were also doing well: already they had been able to leave Lucky once for a couple of hours with no howling. Even better, it had taken about the same time for their granddaughter to settle down to a more relaxed routine at night!

Finally Bibi appeared with Mary. Bibi had got on like a house on fire with Tootsie, the new dog, and within a few days they were to be found cuddled up in the same large dog bed at night and during the afternoons after the morning walk. Actually, this was the cause of the problem now because the walks had turned into gallops with the dogs chasing round the park, jumping and twisting and turning and generally having a marvellous time. After a week of it Bibi had become very stiff and could hardly move. She certainly couldn't keep up with Tootsie.

Mary put Bibi on the table, watched anxiously by Tootsie, who evidently knew that something was wrong. It was quickly obvious what it was: it was general muscular stiffness and soreness. Bibi flinched every time I squeezed any of the muscles in her legs. In short, she was just unfit and unaccustomed to hard exercise. Her appetite had increased in leaps and bounds too. I was amused, and instantly thought back to when I started squad training at Crystal Palace under the discipline of a tough coach. Ten of us were put through our paces, constantly running flat out over 300 metres with ninety seconds' rest between each run. An hour of this was followed by an hour's circuit training. Two days later I had painful abdominal muscles, could hardly straighten up and found walking agonizing. Always the hypochondriac, I was sure I had the early symptoms of appendicitis. I decided to call off the next training session but struggled down to the centre to apologize to the coach. On arrival I saw nine other budding athletes all with the same strained look as me and walking stiffly!

There was no need for Bibi to be in training – there were no races for her to win – but some degree of moderation would be in order until her fitness built up. So it was exercise on the lead for the pair of them with gradually increasing times off it. It was great to see how well they were getting on, playing and wrestling with each other. They were full of the joys of living – and it was a special bonus for Bibi: her mum had always been dominant and had not tolerated too much larking about before giving her daughter a nip. Yet Bibi's pining had been the most severe I have seen – who says animals don't have feelings?

Conditions in humans that potentially cause emotional upset also occur in animals but, of course, the mental suffering is not usually such a problem. Toby, a white Persian cat, had feline acne, which is unlike the condition in dogs and humans. I see only a few cases each year in either dogs or cats and Toby was the first cat acne. Unlike acne in dogs, in cats it is not a deep pus condition. It shows more as a dirty chin. Little blackheads appear, which wouldn't be noticed in the majority of cases except by the most observant of owners. In a brilliant white cat like Toby, however, you couldn't really miss it. The whole of his lower chin was a black greasy spot rather like the neck of a child who refuses to wash! And, funnily enough, in cats that is the key to the problem. Unlike dogs and humans, in which there is a clear relationship with sex hormones, in the cat it appears that acne results from a failure to wash the chin properly. A cat might stop washing and grooming itself for many different reasons, but if the blackheads on the chin become ingrained, help will be needed to sort things out. Toby had had fleas for

96

some time, his skin had become itchy and greasy, and he had been miserable. With the irritation he was grumpy, too, and refused to allow his owner, Gwen, to brush or comb him. In fact, he hadn't been brought in for his acne but for the large knots accumulating in his fur. I would need to administer an anaesthetic before I clipped them out.

I pointed out his dirty, greasy chin. 'I hadn't noticed it, but to tell you the truth he's been such a little devil I've hardly been able to touch him for weeks,' said Gwen. His flea problem had been brought under control with insecticides and now we were faced with getting the fur back in condition and cleaning up his chin. It shouldn't be difficult, I told his owner. First we would clip him out, then give him an injection to reduce inflammation in the skin, continue the flea treatment, and prescribe antibiotics to clear up infection in the chin. Once it was all under control, he could have a little shampooing of the chin when he was more relaxed. Later that day, when Gwen picked up her cat after the first phase of treatment, she was amused to see that Toby's shampoo contained similar ingredients to an acne wash her adolescent son was using. The idea of the special shampoo was to flush the hair follicles, thus clearing the blackheads. Once they had gone Toby might need his chin cleaned regularly to keep them at bay. The things cat owners have to go through!

Keeping an animal happy and healthy is one of the great pleasures of animal ownership – or, at least, it should be – and part of that is to ensure that there is no suffering at the end of a pet's life. This aspect of keeping a pet is one of the hardest. In fact, you could say that by taking on a pet you can expect some heartache when the time comes to say goodbye. We were reaching that stage with old Tom. His owner, Joe, had lived on his own since the death of his wife a few years ago, and the old cat, now approaching fifteen, had been a great source of comfort to him. Having to care for the cat had kept him going. Tom had always been his cat anyway, always choosing to sit on his lap and not his wife's. Whenever anyone visited, Tom would make himself scarce. He was a one-person cat and that was that.

Living a quiet life, with regular vaccinations, spending every night in, he had never had a day's illness until six months ago when he picked up a respiratory infection. Joe had put this down to his new neighbours, who had six cats. Two were unneutered toms, which made him suspect that the owners weren't bothered about their pets. Three weeks ago, Tom had suddenly become ill. He had developed a fever and gone off his food. He had lost weight rapidly and his abdomen had swelled. I had seen the cat and found the swelling to consist of fluid. This condition is called ascites or, to give it a common name, dropsy.

In cats like Tim we have a standard way of investigating the cause. First, a sample of the fluid is tapped from the abdomen and the specific gravity is measured. Tom had quite concentrated fluid. A blood sample is taken to check the liver, kidneys and the amount of protein in the blood. Frequently by the time these results are to hand, we will have a good idea of the problem. It was likely that Tom had viral peritonitis. This is, unfortunately, a fatal condition, which we see fairly regularly. The actual virus is called *coronavirus* and I wanted to send a blood sample to check for evidence of Tom's exposure to it. Apart from the last six months he had not had much contact with other cats. In the meantime, I had given him some pills to try to get rid of the excess fluid and a steroid injection to try to build him up. But it was to no avail. A week later I was going over the latest blood-sample results with Joe. They showed that Tom

had high levels of antibody to the virus, indicating exposure. There was no doubt about the diagnosis and also the
sad fact that the old cat was dying from the disease.

'The only fortunate thing, Joe,' I said, trying to comfort
him, 'is that he isn't in any pain and has lived a very long
life without any illness.' It was true, and if it hadn't been
this problem it would have been something else. It's just
Nature's way when animals become old and the immune
system runs down.

Joe had brought his daughter with him for moral support. Between them they decided to have Tom at home for
the weekend to say goodbye and to make a fuss of him.
Then, on the following Monday, he would have an injection
to put him to sleep. I couldn't offer any effective treatment
apart from trying to keep him comfortable. He had lost
more weight and was hardly eating. Once the diagnosis of
feline viral peritonitis is made, the course of the disease is
usually quick – a matter of weeks.

Mrs Fortuna turned up on the last afternoon consulting
session of the month with four patients, Mr Harry plus three
cats. It was a busy session, and I had just opened my mouth
to ask why she had four animals with her when everyone
else had only one or two, when she got in first.

'Mr Harry's along for the ride. I like to get him used to
the vet so he knows there's nothing to worry about.' I
couldn't argue with that. 'And two of the cats have got the
same thing wrong with them, so it's really only two
patients,' she said.

One had snuffles and sneezing and the other two – one
patient, by Mrs Fortuna's reckoning – had diarrhoea.

'How many cats have you got altogether?' I asked. I'd
always wondered.

'Too many, you'd say,' she said evasively. 'People keep

bringing them to me and I can't not take them in.'

Both the diarrhoea cats were put on a light diet – fish and chicken with rice – to see if a simple measure would sort out the problem. Most virus diseases just need nursing until the body builds up its own resistance. The sneezy cat probably had a virus, too, but would need antibiotics to prevent infection getting into the nasal passages and sinuses. It was a typical case of cat flu, which is rarely fatal but may leave the cat with long-term problems.

Throughout the proceedings Mr Harry sat impassively in the corner of the room. Occasionally one of his eyes would flick up, stare at me, then flick down. He was watching me all the time. The curious thing was his reaction when we got to the snuffly cat. He jumped up, whining, and tried to get on to the table.

'She's his favourite,' Mrs Fortuna explained.

'What? You mean that, of all your cats, this one sticks out in his mind somehow?'

Apparently this was so. Mr Harry had been protective of the cat since she was rescued a few weeks before and she had taken to sleeping in his bed with him.

'And the best of it is,' said Mrs Fortuna, 'I haven't even thought of a name for her yet.'

'How about Henrietta?' I suggested. I was astonished that Mr Harry, living in a house full of cats, should pick just this one to protect. And yet, for whatever reason, they were clearly the best of friends.

JULY

The month opened with a return visit from Butch, the dog with Cushing's disease. Gabriel had admitted him for the first part of the treatment: a drug toxic to the cells in the adrenal gland that are producing too much cortisone. At first it is given every day and always in the hospital, as it is quite a dangerous drug if care is not taken. As these dogs are nearly always drinking too much we measure how much they are consuming and give the drug until the drinking gets back to normal. Once that happens, the dog can be sent home and then the drug need only be given once weekly. Thinking back, I remember seeing a rather forlorn Butch in his kennel: he had never been away from his folks before.

So now I was seeing him for the first time since the treatment had started three months ago, to assess the results. There before me was a changed Butch: hair was growing through everywhere like spring grass; gone was the pot belly, replaced with the physique of a much younger dog; Butch had regained his zest for life. He was dragging his owners around the park instead of the other way round. The drug would have to be given for the rest of his life, and at thirteen we couldn't say how long that might be, but I felt happy that Butch would live a normal life and in all probability it wouldn't be Cushing's disease that ended it.

From a thirteen-year-old crossbreed terrier I went on to my next patient, a year-old Yorkshire terrier. Pip was a poor specimen for his breed, small, underweight and timid. I like Yorkshire terriers – they have tremendous characters and are great extroverts. Not Pip. Small though he was, he tried to make himself even smaller on the consulting table. Maybe it was his owner who intimidated him – he certainly did me at first. Jake was a strapping six-foot plus young man. His hair was so short you couldn't see a parting and his neck and shoulders were as one. It's a funny thing but when I was a student long hair was considered a disgrace – at least, at the veterinary college – but nowadays very short hair is seen as threatening. Together Pip and Jake made quite a contrast, but it was soon apparent that Jake cared deeply for the poor little dog.

'He's been nervous like this ever since we took him on,' he observed sadly. 'I told the wife to pick one of the others in the litter but it was this one she felt sorry for. He wouldn't go out of the house for the first six months. Now he will – but only with the wife. If I take him out he puts the brakes on and I end up carrying him.'

Just as well, I thought. It would be rather comical to see the tiny dog on a lead next to his gentle giant of an owner. As if reading my mind, Jake said, 'Mind you, I don't half get the mick taken by my mates when they see me with the dog! I don't care, though – he's a good little house dog when he's indoors.'

'So what can we do for him?' I asked, but as if to tell me himself the dog started to paw at his mouth. A quick look inside and it was obvious what the problem was. Pip had quite a few extra milk teeth, which should have come out when the permanent teeth erupted at five months of age – quite common in young dogs. Now bits of food and hair were continually getting stuck between his front teeth especially. He wasn't having any trouble eating but every now and then he would paw at his mouth to try to remove whatever was stuck.

Jake had guessed as much, but his wife was terrified of anaesthetics and couldn't bear the thought of something going wrong. She couldn't even bring herself to come to the clinic with her dog. I could understand that: deaths, although rare, do sometimes occur when an animal has been anaesthetized. But anaesthetics now are as safe as they ever have been and the risk is really very small.

With the afternoon list looking quiet, Pip was admitted for the operation that day. It was done by Helen, who reported no problems. Pip had had a cocktail of drugs designed to make him sleepy and to ensure that when he woke up he wouldn't be in pain. Extracting the excess teeth took a mere ten minutes and after another ten Pip was coming round, no doubt wondering what had happened. I am sure, with modern sedative drugs and anaesthetic techniques, that the vast majority of animals suffer little pain and anguish – which is as we like it.

By five-thirty Pip's owners were picking him up. As soon as Pip saw Jake's petite wife, he perked up and settled into her arms. There would be no need for any check-ups. Looking out of my secretary's office window, I watched him being carried to the car, looking a bit sleepy but thoroughly happy. We got a card a few days later, saying how grateful the family were and Pip, too, of course.

It's not just dogs and cats who need their teeth checked. As they get older most animals become prone to tooth problems. In the wild, this is probably a major cause of older animals failing to survive. Recently I came across an interesting article with lovely illustrations about rabbits and their teeth. It turns out that rabbits experience lots of tooth problems and one of the most important causes is low calcium due to their feeding habits. In an hour's reading I learned that if they are fed a mix of cereals and pellets with inadequate greens and hay they tend to leave the pellets, which contain the added calcium, and eat the most tasty mix, which doesn't contain enough calcium, so over a period of time their bones become soft. When this happens in the skull it causes tooth problems. Rabbit teeth, as in all rodents, grow continually and wear against each other. As a consequence of the softened bone, the wearing becomes uneven and either the teeth develop sharp points and may rub against the tongue, or their roots push up or down too far. The upwardly growing tooth roots may interfere with the duct that takes tears from the eye to the nose, and the downward roots start to grow through the jaw-bone. I learned, therefore, that I had to look out for eye problems and drooling due to a painful tongue.

Within a few days of reading this article, I found myself confronted by a rabbit with tooth problems and, for the first time, really felt I understood what was going on – I've lost count of the number of lectures I have been to during which I have picked up on something new only to see it in real life on the following Monday morning! Molly, an eight-year-old rabbit, had come in because she was having difficulty eating hard food. When I examined her jaw I could feel the early signs of tooth roots coming through. She had watery eyes too, and when I talked to Tracey, her owner, who was the same age as her rabbit, I was intrigued to hear that Molly had tended of late not to eat her pellets. It all looked classic for calcium deficiency but to prove it I would need to take an X-ray to check the position of the tooth roots. Under the anaesthetic I could look at the molars too and file them if they were rubbing on Molly's tongue. But anaesthesia would be necessary, and as an eight-year-old rabbit was near its expected normal life-span I felt that it was better to treat Molly with extra calcium and see if she improved. Tracey was relieved about that decision – even at eight she knew about the risks of anaesthetics. On the way out she announced that she wanted to be a vet when she grew up. They start even younger, these days!

I was somewhat surprised to see Joe and his daughter in the afternoon clinic. They had had to say goodbye to Tom the previous day and Joe had decided that he didn't want to be without a cat. The same afternoon they had gone to one of our homing centres and taken on an adult tabby. Now Joe wanted us to give his cat the once-over. To my astonishment one of the nurses immediately recognized it. It had come in with a broken jaw, which had been fixed and the cat nursed back to health. Now neutered, fully vaccinated, microchipped and, like most adult cats, house-trained, he represented a bargain in my eyes. A lovely-natured cat, too.

Joe explained that he and his daughter had had long talks over the weekend. The net result was that he had been persuaded to go and live with her and her family in Norfolk, on condition, of course, that he took a cat with him. The house in Norfolk was huge, and Joe was not happy living on his own. Moving to Norfolk would benefit everyone – not least Tom, as the tabby had been called. Two of the nurses who had spent hours feeding Tom by tube, and later with a syringe, were delighted to see a complete change in his fortunes. The trouble with nursing stray cats back to health is that we so rarely hear the end of the story, and we always wonder whether they finally made it to a caring home. Tom certainly had.

The rain plummeted down. It was the Wimbledon finals and poor old Jeremy had organized a day off to see the tennis. No such luck – it was rained off. But this kind of weather is tricky: we sometimes see heatstroke on days like this when an unsuspecting owner leaves their dog in the car in the middle of a heavy shower only to find that it was *just* a shower. In a matter of minutes when the sun has come out the car is an oven and the dog may die. The only safe thing to do in the heat of summer is never to leave animals unattended in the car. Even this advice can backfire: with everyone travelling to the coast on hot days, traffic jams can easily build up and the family pet can suffer heatstroke even with everyone on board. My old dog Barney used to sit between my passenger's legs on hot days with the fan blowing full blast. I have also seen heatstroke in dogs who have been tied up in the garden, so it doesn't only happen in cars. But cars are perhaps the highest profile cause of the problem and every year at Wimbledon the RSPCA inspectors are at hand to check the car-parks. It seems, though, that this is one animal-welfare message that is getting across because the numbers of heatstroke victims are decreasing, at least in my experience, and fortunately we hadn't seen one yet this year.

The sun can cause damage in other ways, too. Over the last twenty years there has been an increase in animal skin cancer. This may be due partly to the fact that animals are living longer and perhaps also to the damage to the ozone layer. Skin cancer, in both animals and people, is no longer only seen in sunny places like Australia and California: in the UK, in cats, sun-induced skin cancer is now the commonest type I see. All the more pleasing, therefore, to see a case in a cat that had not actually reached the malignant stage. If caught early, the cancer is curable, but the surgery is quite radical. Since the affected part of the body is usually the ears, they have to be removed.

Bianca was an old cat in the earliest stage of the disease.

She was thirteen – a typical age to develop skin cancer – and her owner, Miss Renwick, had been quick to detect the subtle changes in her cat. As befits her name, Bianca was almost entirely white – it's always white cats or white bits of cats that have sun-induced problems. The tips of her ears had become reddened and slightly curled and Miss Renwick was worried that it might be the early stage of skin cancer. While chatting to her I found out that, at the age of seventy-five, she had just finished a basic science degree at the Open University – small wonder that she had been so quick to think of sun damage.

I felt reasonably sure that Bianca was not at the cancerous stage – the squamous cell carcinoma, as it is called. Before this happens, there is normally a period in which the sun causes inflammation and skin damage, solar dermatitis, which is treatable without disfiguring surgery. I discussed the issues with the sprightly Miss Renwick. Of course, simply taking off the tops of Bianca's ears would cure her because the hair further down would protect the remainder of the ear from further damage. On the other hand, Bianca had had kidney disease and might not be a very good anaesthetic risk. We agreed on a plan. Bianca would have a course of steroids to reduce the inflammation. She would not be allowed out between the hours of nine a.m. and three p.m. when the sun is at its hottest and, even in the house, she would not be allowed to bask by the windows. Ultraviolet light can still damage skin through window-panes. It didn't surprise me to discover that Bianca was a sun-worshipper, as have been virtually all the cats I have seen with this disease. There was one thing further we could do and that was to put sun-block factor 30 on the tips of her ears each morning on sunny days. This may seem a bizarre thing to do to a cat but it is entirely sensible. It can also be put on other vulnerable sites, such as the nose and the lower eyelids. If distracted for five minutes the cat will leave the sun-block alone and be protected from damage. By the laws of average, we were due for a sunny, hot spell and we could monitor how things went over the next few weeks.

Miss Renwick left the clinic, happy that we had avoided the trauma of surgery for the time being. She was going to read up on sun-induced cancers, ultraviolet light and the ozone layer. I looked forward to being educated next time she was in!

A few days later, we were well into summer with the usual glut of problems that brings. On ward rounds, after a particularly hot day, there were four cats who had fallen from high-rise balconies; we had a very busy morning surgery with lots of itchy dogs and cats; and on the prep room list there were several dogs with grass seeds in their paws. At this time of year we have to be extra careful, too, with any animal with an eye infection. Panda, a fluffy young cat, had been seen a few days earlier with apparent conjunctivitis. She had a very swollen eye – so swollen it was difficult to see anything. She had been given some eye ointment to reduce the inflammation, and her owner had been asked to come back in a day or so if there was no improvement. Now, two days later, she was back and just visible at the corner of the eye was the telltale stalk of a grass seed. With a gentle tug it was out. I could now expect a complete cure within a week, but I was left thinking how easy it could have been for the grass seed to stay in for much longer and with disastrous consequences.

The same morning a spaniel came in with a swollen paw. I knew it would be a grass seed – the signs are so typical – and I was just about to admit him for an anaesthetic and to search for the seed when I caught sight of a small stalk right in the corner of the space between the claws. A quick tug and out came a seed. Great! Problem solved and cage space kept open. Recently I had been caught unawares by a sudden run on dog kennels – we had been inundated by a larger than usual number of emergencies. The reports nurse was already busy phoning all the owners of dogs who could possibly go home to try to get them out early.

I spent my lunch-hour trying to catch up on my reading. My system is to put all articles and journals on the left side of my desk. As they get read I put them into the filing system with the aim of having nothing on the desk, although that hardly ever happens. The truth is that it is practically impossible to get on top of all the developments in veterinary medicine. That is the benefit of having colleagues, and it seems to me that that is where the future lies. Individual practices will have specialists in most areas on site or smaller practices will send all complicated cases to centres where detailed investigations can be made. In our hospital there is a natural gravitation towards individual expertise, which makes keeping up to date easier: we all update each other almost automatically. The striking thing, however, is that although there is much professional enjoyment to be had from the latest scientific developments and their application there is still, at least for me, just as much enjoyment in simple cases and cures.

After a working lunch grappling with the complexities of how to treat fractures that have failed to heal, and an article on every conceivable aspect of ringworm, then a learned treatise on nervous diseases, which I found very difficult to understand, my first case of the afternoon was Jo-Jo. An eighteen-year-old tabby cat, she had suddenly gone lame on her right front leg and the paw had swollen. She couldn't bear it to be touched. The demeanour of both Jenny Smith and her mother, Susan, indicated that they feared the worst. When any old animal has an apparently severe illness, the thoughts of the owners inevitably stray to the idea that their pet might be suffering from cancer. In an eighteen-year-old cat that would probably be very serious, and Susan, in particular, had made up her mind that Jo-Jo had come to the end of the line.

'She just suddenly went lame,' Susan said, as soon as Jo-Jo was on the table, 'and we're worried she's got bone cancer.'

Cancer of the bone is not common in cats, though, and I set about the usual methodical way of examining any lame animal. We usually start at the paw and work up. The paw was obviously swollen and very painful. Like most very old cats, Jo-Jo made a great fuss when she was examined, including bloodcurdling shrieks, which would have deterred any feline antagonist but which, for once, were not accompanied by any physical attacks on me. Almost immediately the cause of the acute lameness popped up. With increasing age, Jo-Jo had taken to sleeping the greater part of her time and didn't go out much. Certainly she didn't sharpen her claws much. It would have been easy to miss, just like the grass seed in Panda's eye. But there it was: a claw had grown right into the pad and had developed an infection. It was concealed by hair but just at the corner I could see a little blood seeping from where the claw had penetrated.

'Hold tight!' I told Susan and her daughter. 'She'll feel this but she'll be free of pain straight away afterwards.'

Gently holding Jo-Jo's paw and pulling back the fur, I could see the claw curving right into her flesh. With a quick snip I cut the claw right back and pulled it out of the pad. There was a loud hiss as Jo-Jo tried to scratch me and then

110

she went quiet. All that was necessary now was an injection of antibiotic, some tablets, and she could go home cured. As though to prove the point, she scampered back into her basket – on four paws. For Jenny and Susan it was a transition from deep foreboding to happiness. Jo-Jo's time hadn't come, after all. Three satisfied customers, and for me a reminder that although it was important to try to keep up to date with the latest developments there was still plenty of satisfaction to be had from the mundane, though Jo-Jo might not have agreed.

By the middle of the month we were still trying to keep the lists quiet and I was doing my best on ward rounds to send home as many animals as I could. As always, one or two owners had left their pets for two or three days longer than necessary and the odd one had been dumped. I have never understood those people who seem concerned and caring when their cat or dog is admitted but who then fail to make any further contact. It would save a lot of hassle if they just said right away that they couldn't cope and then everyone would know what was going on. Still, it wasn't as bad as some weeks: we had to send out only one recorded-delivery letter to remind someone that their kitten with the broken leg was doing well and could go home. Failure to reply to the letter within a week would mean the kitten going to the homing centre, along with all the others. I was gearing up, too, for the really bad time of year for stray cats, which is from now until September when people go on holiday and abandon their pet.

The main reason for trying to keep the operating lists and number of hospitalized animals down was that half a dozen or more of the trainee animal nurses would be taking their exams. It takes at least two years to qualify as an animal nurse. At the end of each year there is a written examination, which is pretty tough, followed by practical exams. We had first- and second-year trainees swotting like mad and, of course, they needed time off to sit the exams. Most had also arranged some annual leave so that they could spend all day revising. The practical training goes on during their day-to-day work but they also attend theory lectures at various colleges in London. Once they have sat the exams they have to wait until August to know the results. I had high hopes from the present bunch as they had all worked hard but we would have to wait and see.

In ward eight I found a couple of chickens, one of which had laid an egg for us. They had been seen running down a high street in the East End the night before and had been caught by the police. Late at night they had been admitted by the night staff, who had bedded them down with some food, and were bemused to see a large egg the next morning. How on earth had two chickens come to be running down a high street in the middle of the night? Stray chickens are common visitors to the hospital but they are never claimed. Somehow we always manage to find somewhere for them to go. The story with these two, although I couldn't verify it, was that they had been seen jumping out of a lorry destined for the slaughterhouse! At least, that was what an anonymous caller phoned in to say later that morning. I wasn't inclined to follow it up and, as luck would have it, we were able to get both into a city farm within a day or so. There they could live out their lives unless the actual owners came to claim them this week. I hoped that wouldn't happen. At least they weren't cockerels again – they are so difficult to place due to the racket they kick up.

Also in ward eight there were several blackbird fledglings, which would need to go to centres specialized in rehabilitation. If we were to release them in our gardens they would almost certainly not survive. It had taken a lot of hard work to get them this far and we were keen to get it right.

The ward was filling up – I had forgotten that it wasn't just cats and dogs which get abandoned at holiday-time but smaller pets, too, who are literally put out in the streets or left on our doorstep. We were back to the same problem we had in June. I counted four hamsters, six rabbits, two mice, a young guinea-pig and two rats, the latter having been dumped in a telephone box. None had owners. All would need innumerable phone calls before we found new homes for them. Somehow we always do – those dedicated nurses again. Often they spend their lunch-breaks phoning round our contacts. With a bit of luck we would clear out the ward so that the emergency crew could concentrate on the sick and injured animals that usually flood in at weekends during the summer months.

Sometimes we can't cure animals but manage to keep them reasonably healthy on permanent medication. I had been treating Eddy, a twelve-year-old English bull terrier, for more than five years without ever getting to the real cause of his problem. This breed is prone to skin ailments, particularly allergies. Duchess, who figured prominently on a previous series of *Animal Hospital*, was a classic example, and we eventually got her under good control with shampoos and high doses of evening-primrose oil. This was a bit of luck because not all allergies respond to this treatment.

Eddy had the other problem that seems to crop up in the breed: he had suddenly developed infection in the skin of his legs. I had isolated the germ that was causing it and put him on antibiotics. A month later he seemed to be cured, but within a few weeks of stopping the antibiotics the deep infection was back. This did not surprise me because it's a well-known fact that infections of this sort usually have an

113

underlying cause – but what was it? This question exercised my mind for the following year. Eddy was skin-scraped in case he had mites, he was tested for Cushing's disease (like Butch) and for an inactive thyroid gland. It didn't matter what I tested him for, though, as the results came back relentlessly as normal. In the end, I had to admit defeat and keep the dog on more or less permanent antibiotics. I tried three months on then a month off, high dose, normal dose and low dose, and eventually we found that most of the time Eddy lived a normal life on one pill a day. We had occasional flare-ups, which always responded to a higher dose of four pills a day. A lot of people will throw up their hands in despair at using antibiotics in this way and look for alternative remedies, but it is a textbook method of treating these animals. Eddy's family were sensible too, and as long as the dog didn't seem to be suffering any side-effects they were happy that we had found a way to keep him normal. One thing I was certain of: if we stopped the antibiotics his skin would flare up within a couple of weeks. I hadn't been able to prove it but I assumed that there was a defect with Eddy's skin immune system, which allowed these infections to take hold.

But today he was in for something else. A quick check-up of his skin showed a few scars where the deepest part of the infection had been, but it was his nose that I was concerned with. English bull terriers have fine large noses, and on the end of Eddy's was a nasty-looking growth. It had come up in a matter of days and was some kind of skin cancer. Things like this are common in old dogs and cats, and Eddy was old, with a suspect immune system.

His family had obviously had a long chat before they arrived at the hospital. Was this the end of the road? they asked. From a surgical point of view, the growth looked

114

removable. It would all depend on which type of cancer we were dealing with. A few days later, the old dog was in the operating theatre. A very gentle animal, he had submitted to the needle going into his vein with the quiet resignation of a placid dog who has seen a lot of the vet in his time. Half an hour later he had eight stitches in his nose and the growth was on its way to the histopathologist who would analyse it for me. We would now have to wait. Within a few hours the family arrived to take him home. Eddy plodded off as though this was part of his normal routine. Not for him the anguish I might feel if I was waiting for the result of a potentially very serious condition. He was just happy to be on his way home.

A couple of days later I found myself examining a billy goat. When was the last time I had treated one? I wondered. Probably around 1971. I had thought my goat days were over. Not so – for there in the run between wards seven and eight was a large and apparently un-named and perfect specimen of Billy goat. Not only that, he was tremendously friendly and loved having his ears tickled. He had been admitted first thing on Sunday morning and I was told he had fallen thirty feet on to a railway track. I checked him over and couldn't find a thing wrong with him. Nonchalantly munching some hay provided by the nurses and looking thoroughly contented with all the attention he was attracting, it seemed he was content to stay with us. Later that day Ned, the ambulance driver who had rescued him, filled me in with all the details.

The goat was owned by a Mr Austin, who had several. Our patient had strayed on to a viaduct over a disused railway line and somehow managed to fall off. The ground under the viaduct was a favourite site for car-boot sales and it was when the organizers had arrived early on Sunday to set up that they had found Billy roaming around, slightly disoriented. A call to the RSPCA resulted in Ned being dispatched to bring him back to the hospital for a check-up. The goat's owner was known to the inspectors and he was informed of the whereabouts of his animal. I'm quite sure he was due for a lecture on making sure that his grazing ground was secure. Looking at Billy, I found it hard to believe that he had survived such a fall unscathed. The other thing that struck me was how relaxed he was – he was obviously used to a lot of contact with friendly people. My recollection of goats was that they could sometimes bite – and feeling his rather sharp horns I didn't fancy a head-butt either. Now Mr Austin would have to arrange transport home for him and I anticipated daily phone calls to remind him. The nurses were quite happy to keep Billy and I could see why these lovely creatures so often end up as regimental mascots – if I wasn't careful I'd have a hospital mascot on my hands! In fact, after three or four reminders Mr Austin came and took Billy home. We were all sad to see him go.

Right at the end of the week I heard the telltale high-pitched shriek indicating that a fax was on its way in. I was about to go home but waited to see if it was anything interesting. It was: Eddy's growth was benign and, according to the histopathologist, it had all come out. What a relief to his owners. There was life in the old dog yet! It was excellent news all round because the next day I was off to a cottage on the Northumberland coast. I was looking forward to a gathering of the Grant family and it was great to go away knowing that Eddy would be okay.

AUGUST

August is always a busy month, along with September. I think of it as a time dominated by allergies and, without doubt, fleas account for most of them. For one reason or another, and I have never been able to fathom it out completely, the onset of the annual flea epidemic occurs around 10 August when we suddenly see a huge increase in the numbers of people coming to the clinic. Quite often it occurs after a warm weekend and on Monday morning queues develop early. By the end of the day we will have seen getting on for two hundred patients, if we include the two satellite clinics.

We see dogs and cats in about equal numbers, most with skin disease. To the vet the diagnosis is obvious but it never is to the owner. During each day, for some six weeks until the onset of colder weather, consultation after consultation is characterized by every human response from incredulity, shock, anger, embarrassment – and occasionally acceptance of the diagnosis! Although flea allergy is obvious to any vet with experience, most owners know little about fleas. Because the animal is itchy, any evidence of the insects is usually licked or scratched off, so the owner will not generally believe the diagnosis.

A slightly different case was a mother cat and her litter of three kittens, who had been admitted as an emergency. Miss Marples, an old lady who lived on her own, was the owner of Sophie, who was struggling to bring up her first litter even though she wasn't yet a year old. Three weeks ago she had had six kittens and took to them straight away, in spite of being so young. Then, one by one, three had faded away and died. When the fourth kitten began to ail Miss Marples came along at nine one evening to see what, if anything, could be done. I was still there catching up on paperwork but I needn't have worried about the diagnosis as the duty nurse, Jackie, already felt she knew. She phoned up to my office and said, 'I think we've got a case of flea anaemia.' I went down to the prep room where I was confronted by a thin, slightly scruffy-looking cat with three even thinner, sleepy kittens. The mother cat had a musty odour about her and didn't respond to anything.

'How many cats has Miss Marples got now?' I asked Jackie.

'Loads, I think,' was the answer.

Certainly she was a familiar enough figure in the hospital and she lived for her cats, although no one had been able to find out how many she had. Apparently she was known in the area as a cat lover and people would sometimes bring cats to her. Occasionally she would find homes for a few, but more often than not she couldn't bear to be parted from them and they would just become part of her extended family. I suppose that was the key to it: without them she would have been very lonely. As far as I knew she had never married and had no immediate family, although she never divulged the slightest bit of information about herself apart from being a cat lover. Having seen her on quite a few occasions I never got to know her any more than just her surname.

Apart from being thin Sophie was in reasonable condition. That was another thing about Miss Marples: hard though it must be for a pensioner to find the money to feed

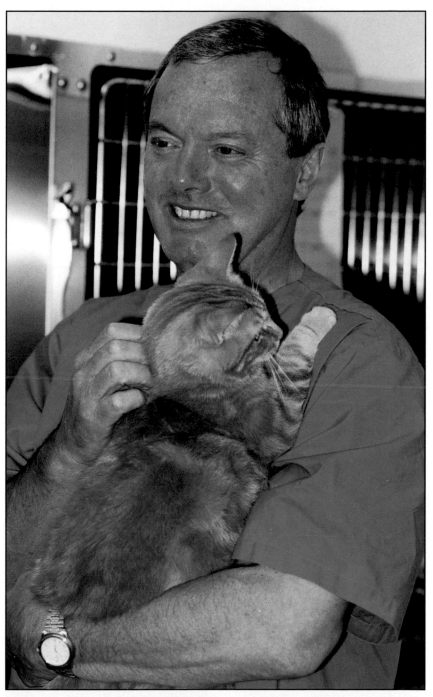

In the isolation ward, this stray cat had just recovered from flu. He was a big favourite of mine and all the nurses.
(© Zara Napier)

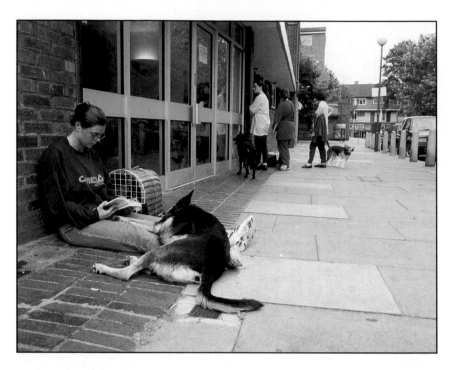

The waiting room at the Harmsworth can get pretty busy.
On sunny days owners often sit outside. (© Zara Napier)

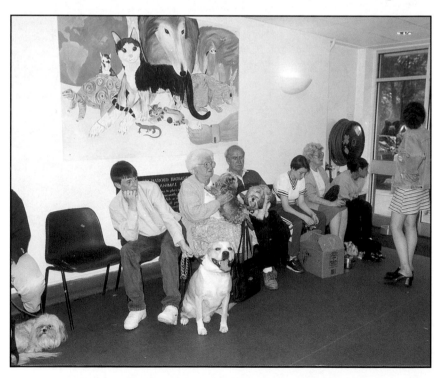

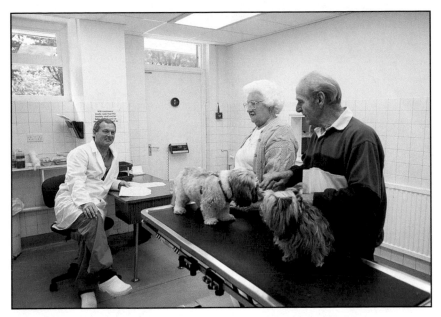

A lot of dogs are well behaved on the examining table.
This pair didn't seem to mind too much. (© Zara Napier)

But I don't like to take a chancc with the larger dogs. This
poor chap's eyes are very expressive and you can tell he's
not looking forward to what comes next. (© Zara Napier)

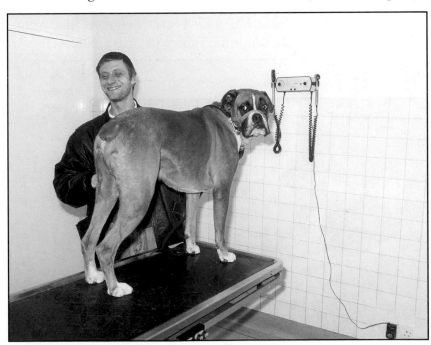

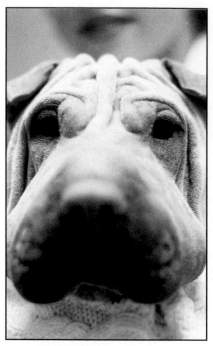

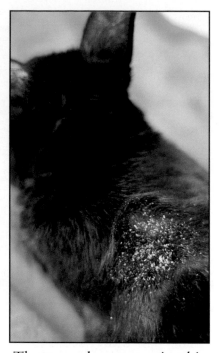

This year I saw three Sharpeis. This is Shannon, who was stung on the nose by a bee. (© David Grant)

Thumper demonstrating his bad case of dandruff, one indication of his mite infestation. (© David Grant)

This beautiful white cat was a lot better behaved than some I've had on the examining table. (© Zara Napier)

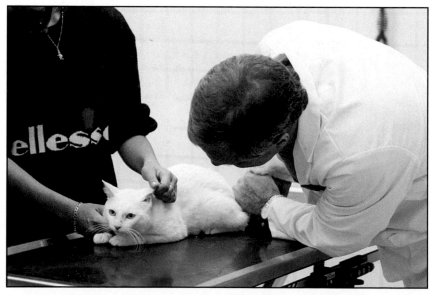

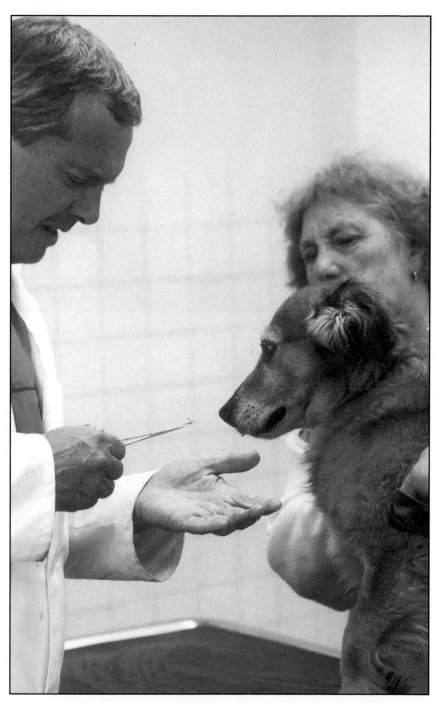

Sam was relieved to have the grass seed removed from his
paw. It's a common problem in the summer months.
(© Zara Napier)

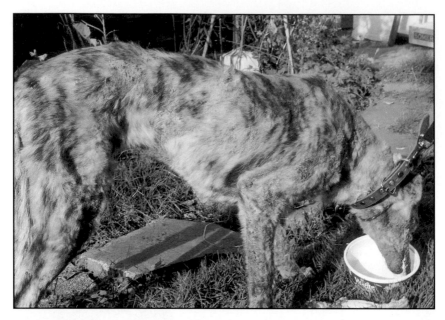

Greyhound Heidi soon after she first went home with Phil,
her skin condition still very painful. (© Phil Williams)

Now a fully recovered Heidi is very much one of the family.
(© Zara Napier)

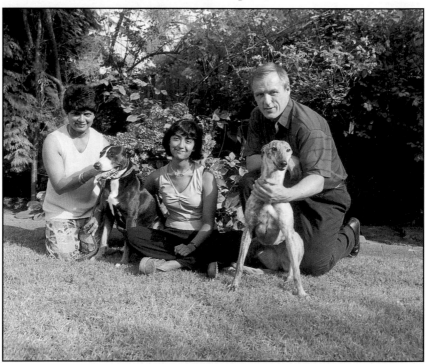

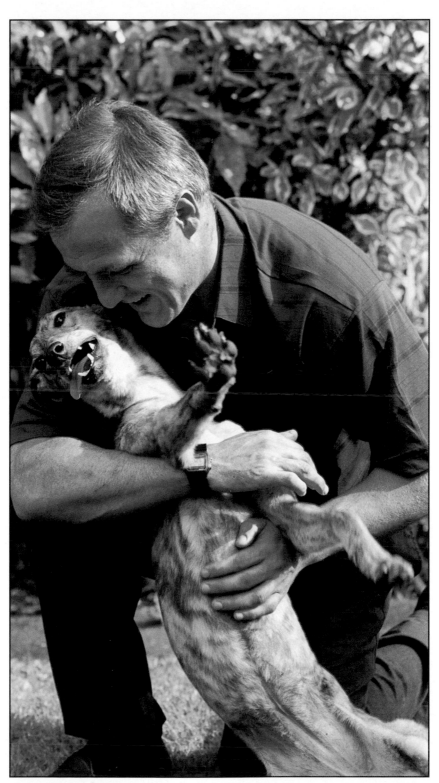

(© Zara Napier)

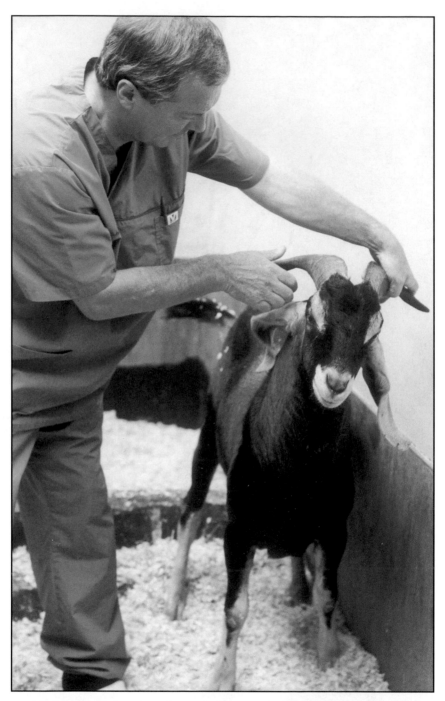

This is Billy, one of our more unusual patients. He fell
thirty feet from a viaduct, but was miraculously unhurt.
(© Zara Napier)

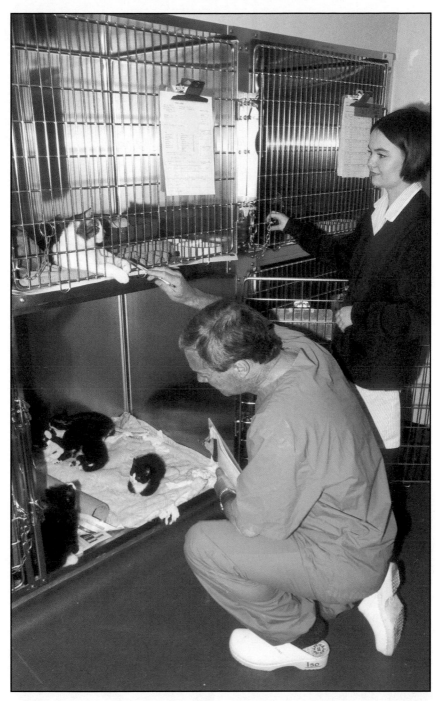

On ward rounds, checking some patients with nurse Emma.
(© Zara Napier)

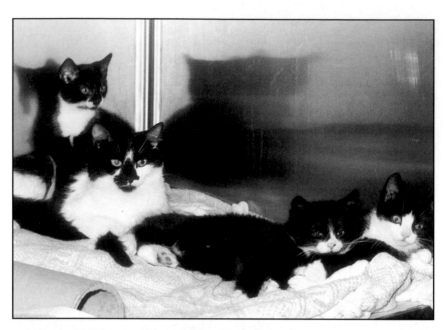

We always have plenty of stray cats – this mother and her
three kittens are doing well.
(© Zara Napier)

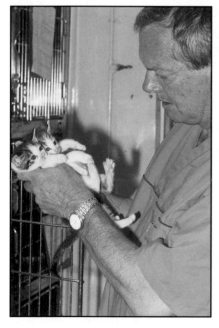

These two strays are only six
weeks old.
(© Zara Napier)

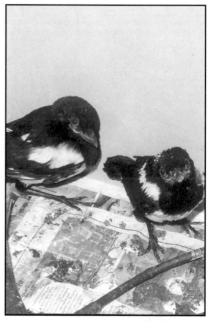

Kept well away from the cats
are these magpie fledglings.
(© Zara Napier)

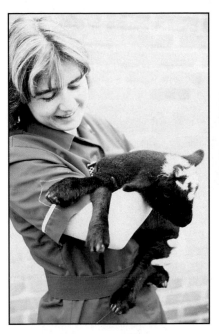

This lamb was found on a
train in the East End. Lizzie,
like all the nurses, fell in
love with her.

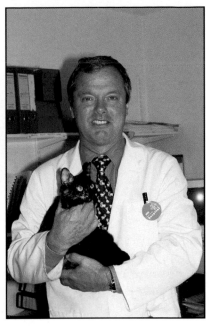

Lottie fell 200 feet from a
high rise balcony – and was
perfectly all right.
(© David Grant)

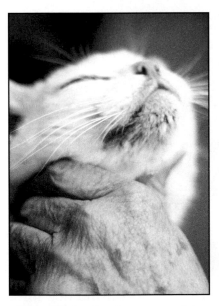

Poor Toby had acne on his
chin – yes, cats can get it too.
(© David Grant)

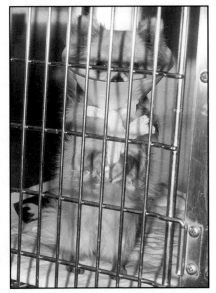

A lot of dogs have to wear
these Elizabethan collars. Not
surprisingly, they don't like it.
(© Zara Napier)

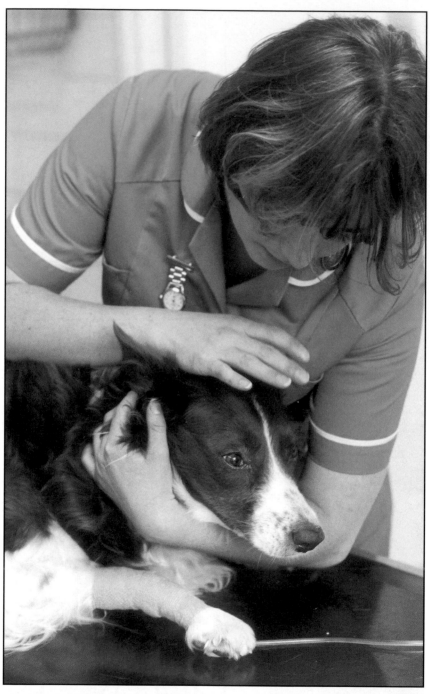

In the prep room Lizzie prepares a twelve-year-old dog for a
hysterectomy.
(© Zara Napier)

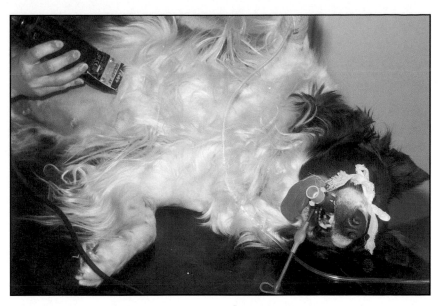

Being shaved for her operation.
(© Zara Napier)

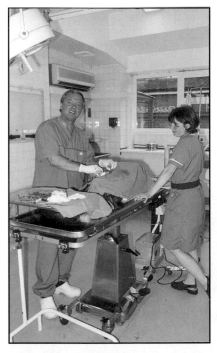

The operation itself is one of
the most common we perform.
(© Zara Napier)

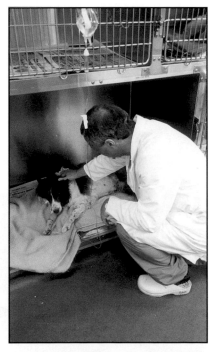

It went well and she was
soon recovering.
(© Zara Napier)

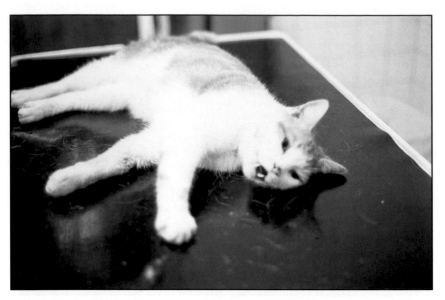

Ginger came in as an emergency, suffering from a severe asthma attack. Lying on the table it was clear he could barely breathe. (©David Grant)

Thankfully we were able to get his condition under control and here he is recovering well. (©David Grant)

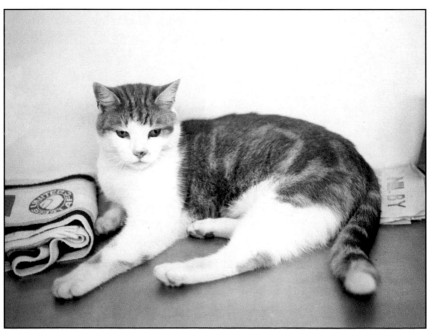

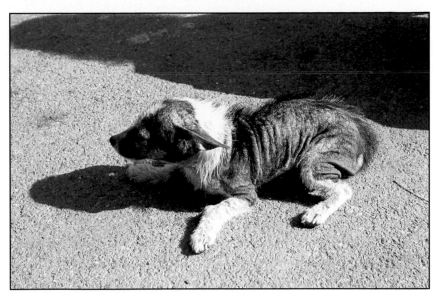

When Scrap was rescued by Bob and his German shepherd Sally the little puppy was suffering from demodectic mange and had virtually no hair. (©David Grant)

Here he is fully recovered. (©David Grant)

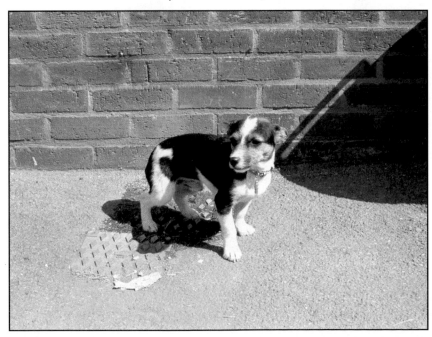

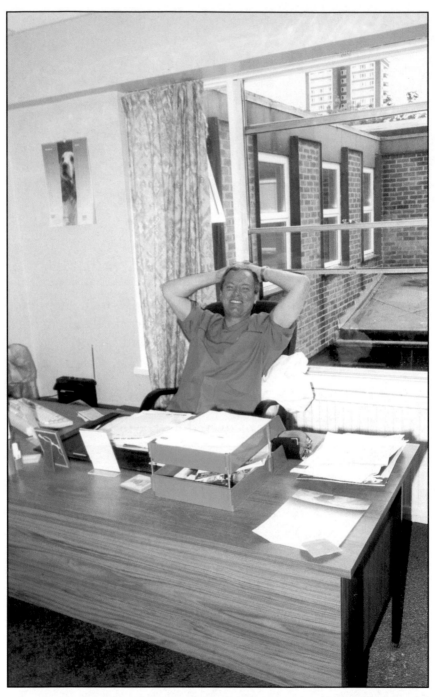

Catching up on some paperwork at the end of the day.
(©Zara Napier)

several cats Miss Marples's were usually in pretty good condition. Multi-cat households, though, throw up their fair share of diseases which its members pass among themselves. They are prone to flea problems. I found quite a lot of fleas on Sophie, and a check of the three kittens showed that Jackie was right – they were all suffering from anaemia. Their tongues and gums were pallid and their hearts were pounding in a frantic attempt to get what blood remained round all the systems. A careful look through the coats of each kitten found a surprisingly large number of fleas – I say surprising because fleas are so adept at hiding. Not in the least surprising that Miss Marples would maintain the next day that she hadn't seen any fleas 'for quite some time'.

Flea larvae depend on blood for them to develop into the next stage – the pupa – although they don't feed on blood directly: they eat their mother's droppings! Female fleas are voracious drinkers of blood: they take far more than they need for themselves and it just passes through their guts unchanged to act as food for their young. At their peak, females can lay fifty eggs a day, which soon produces many hungry mouths to feed. In one day a female flea can drink blood of up to fifteen times her body weight. All this means that young animals, such as kittens and puppies, are vulnerable to developing anaemia if they are allowed to become infested with large numbers of fleas. It is a very common problem for us to have to deal with, especially in long hot summers.

Traditionally we dealt with fleas on kittens by picking them off one by one with a flea comb. Nowadays we have such safe insecticides that we can spray even nursing mums with sickly kittens. A few minutes later Jackie and I had sprayed Sophie, fed her, and picked fleas off the kittens. We gave them all multivitamin injections and, finally, wormed Sophie. Then it was a waiting game to see if the kittens started to pick up. The chances were good – sadly, more so since three kittens had already died and there was more milk available for the survivors. Already dead fleas could be seen dropping away from Sophie. But what about the rest of the cats at home? Here was the real problem and I resolved to leave that one until the morning. It was already gone ten in the evening – time to get home.

The next day I decided to enlist the help of the inspectors. There were several possibilities but it seemed to me that getting the council in (with Miss Marples's permission, of course) to deal with the infestation would be a good thing and then we could treat the adult cats. Veterinary surgeons have access to so many anti-flea products now – we are spoilt for choice – and things are set to improve even further with more in the pipeline. We can attack fleas on at least three fronts, with products to kill the adults, others that make the eggs infertile, and yet more to attack developing fleas in the home. It's definitely not a good time to be a flea. All that is required is a good understanding of the flea life-cycle and the right approach. There would be little point in sending the kittens home until we had Miss Marples's flea problem under control.

The following week, at eight in the evening, I was doing a mini ward round after seeing a few pets in the emergency clinic. Night duties are usually busier in summer but somehow it doesn't seem so bad when it's warm and light. It was Thursday and I was looking forward to the weekend and spending it mostly in the garden, maybe with a barbecue or two.

I was woken from my daydream by Clare, one of the evening's shift nurses. She had just spoken to one of our regular clients whose cat appeared to be dying. His owners were rushing him in. I got out the clinical record card. The cat I was expecting was called Ginger and he was eight. For the last two years he had been treated on and off for asthma, but had never had to come in out of hours. He had had a dry cough, which we had treated in several different ways but without much success. Bairbre had X-rayed his chest, and discovered that Ginger had asthma: the signs were subtle, with overinflation of the lungs and the heart appearing slightly smaller than usual, but to someone like Bairbre, who is experienced in interpreting X-rays, it was pretty conclusive.

I hadn't known much about this condition in cats so I had taken an interest in Ginger. For the last year his problem had been contained to flare-ups, which we managed with injections of steroids. Various attempts had been made to find out the cause but we had had to assume eventually that he was allergic to something, although we didn't know what.

A few minutes later Clare rushed him through. I saw at a glance that he was on his last legs. Lying on his side he was fighting for breath with his tongue lolling out. The most disturbing thing was that the tongue was a dark blue instead of the usual healthy salmon pink. Clare bundled him into an oxygen tent and quickly pumped in 100 per cent oxygen. While she was doing this I made for the emergency box that we always have handy for the rare anaesthetic emergency. In there I found a vial of adrenaline. I snapped it open, filled a syringe and jabbed it into one of Ginger's muscles. Then I drew up two further injections, one of a steroid, another of a drug called millophylline. All these drugs were designed to help relax the bronchial muscles, which are constricted in a severe acute asthmatic attack. I had to assume that this was what was wrong with Ginger, although I had had little time to examine him in any detail. Given the history of intermittent attacks, it was the most likely diagnosis. In any case, if I was right, there might be a dramatic improvement following the emergency treatment.

While Clare monitored his progress in the oxygen tent I popped out to talk to Ginger's owners, two sisters who had lived together for forty years and were now pensioners. They had always had cats and Ginger was the latest in a long line. They had never before experienced anything like this and were blaming themselves. Of course it wasn't their fault and I tried to put their minds at rest.

'We don't actually know a lot about asthma,' I explained, 'and I've never seen anything quite like this myself, but I think Ginger is suffering from *status asthmaticus*.' This rather posh-sounding name refers to the situation that occurs when an animal goes into a severe attack, which gets progressively worse and leads to death unless treated. Nothing different had occurred that day to explain the attack. I went back into the recovery room where Ginger was showing signs of improvement. His breathing attempts were nothing like so frantic and his tongue was pink again. Also, he was trying to sit up. It looked as though Clare and I had saved him, and I went out to tell the sisters that the immediate crisis had passed. The news was greeted with tears of relief and hugs.

I knew exactly how they felt: my elder daughter had suffered her first asthma attack while we were on holiday only a few weeks before. Fortunately, it was nothing like as bad as Ginger's but we took her to hospital so that the attack could be controlled with a nebulizer. Attaching this to an infant's nose was easier said than done! Asthma is increasing dramatically in children and the reason for this is uncertain as far as I know although some people are blaming it on pollution. The Northumberland coast is very clean so it could hardly be the cause in Laura's case. Asthma doesn't seem to be dramatically on the increase in animals unless I am missing the diagnosis, so the real answers are not yet apparent.

The next day on ward rounds Ginger was looking bright and cheerful and tucking into his breakfast. In the calm of the morning I looked through his records again. The only thing we hadn't done was skin-test him to see if we could pinpoint any allergies. He had been on a special diet for six weeks to test for food allergy, which more commonly causes skin disease than asthma in cats, but this hadn't helped. In any case Ginger's problem was intermittent, so food was unlikely. It looked as if he would have to spend some time on steroids as we could not allow another episode like last night's to occur. He had very nearly died. At the present state of knowledge about asthma, it seemed unlikely that I would ever find the true cause of Ginger's condition so control it would have to be, but I didn't feel too bad about this as control not cure is the usual scenario with people.

August, of course, is the prime holiday month and it being a Thursday we were two vets down. Bairbre was on holiday and Gabriel had a couple of days off after working all the previous weekend. Perversely at these times, even though we try to keep the operating lists down, it's apt to become hectic. As I was snatching a cup of tea mid-morning and replying to letters from children who wanted to know about becoming a vet, I was interrupted by Clare, who was again working with me that morning. She telephoned from theatre: there was currently no vet around and a dog had just come in bleeding from the mouth. The owner had been able to tell us the cause – a stick injury.

John Bolton, a man in his forties who had been made redundant six months ago and had been unable to find work since, was out with his dog for his morning walk. He had got the dog from the dogs' home a year ago since having a mild heart attack – the exercise would do him good, his doctor had told him. The dog, a Jack Russell – John had called him Jack – loved nothing more than chasing sticks and bringing them back. Seemingly he could spend all day retrieving them without showing signs of tiring. I remembered John coming to the surgery with Jack soon after getting him. He had been through a rough patch and, as so often happens, came out with the whole story almost immediately.

There wasn't much wrong with his dog – reassurance was all that was needed. This is part of a vet's job which happens a lot. When life is difficult and things go wrong people worry even more about their pets and problems which under normal circumstances might seem relatively minor take on far bigger proportions. Since then, things had certainly improved for John. He had shed a couple of stones, stopped smoking and, with Jack, was doing an hour or two of walking each day. He had high hopes of getting work too.

On learning what had happened to Jack I wasn't too worried. Over the years I have seen quite a lot of stick injuries and most need just a stitch at the back of the throat. Occasionally a sliver of wood detaches itself and migrates through the neck, causing an infection called a sinus. The only cure for this is to find the bit of wood, which can be like looking for a needle in a haystack. I have to admit that throwing sticks was something I used to do for my dog Barney. Even though he could run like the wind in his younger days I always reckoned I could throw it so far that

124

it invariably landed before he reached it. The problem with these sticks is that if the dog catches up with the stick and at the same time it lands vertically it can so easily go into the mouth. Sometimes the stick breaks into two as it lands, leaving a jagged edge. In all probability the same thing had happened to Jack.

In the prep room Clare had set up a drip. I had asked her to do this on the phone before I made my way down. I was impressed as always by her efficiency – it had taken me two minutes at the most to get out of my office and down to the prep room and yet it was ready when I arrived. She had also given the dog his premedication (a painkiller and sedative) as instructed. With these we can give less anaesthetic and the dog will be free of pain when it comes round from the operation.

There was quite a lot of blood round Jack's mouth, which looked alarming, but a check of his gums and tongue showed that it wasn't anything like as bad as it looked. The healthy salmon pink colour showed that he hadn't lost much blood. It never ceases to amaze me how a relatively small amount of blood can make an inordinate amount of mess.

John, who was in a state of near shock, was still in the hospital sitting in a recess of the reception we use for situations like this. Terry the receptionist had got him a cup of tea and I nipped out to speak to him.

'You all right?' I asked. It was a pretty daft question, since he was trembling and very pale. 'Try not to worry,' I said. 'I'm just going to sort Jack out now. It's not as bad as you think. You can stay here if you want and I'll let you know as soon as I'm finished.'

A couple of minutes later, Jack was asleep on the operating table. The wound in the back of his throat was bigger than most but easy to stitch and would heal quickly as there is such a good blood supply in the area. He would go home that evening. That's another feature of August – the hospital is constantly bulging at the seams and we try to get everything home as soon as possible. As soon as he was safely round from his anaesthetic I sent a message to his owner, who was also looking a lot better if feeling a bit guilty. He'd be throwing a rubber bone from now on.

Later on in the afternoon I was reminded of the importance of reassurance for owners when I found myself examining a lugubrious old crossbreed dog with the highly improbable name of Prince Boy. It was a hot August afternoon with a great crowd of animals and their owners. Some were even sunbathing outside while the rest sweated it out in the waiting room. From time to time one of the more impatient owners would ask how much longer they had to wait, and on afternoons like this an hour or so is quite possible. Some people just can't put up with it and the heat brings out the worst in them. So it was with a mild degree of irritation that I looked at Prince Boy's clinical record. Over the last two years he had attended the hospital no fewer than twenty-four times. On most of these occasions nothing much had been wrong: he had a cold, or he wouldn't eat, or was scratching. Nothing else. He had been admitted twice and had had three sets of blood tests. Treatment had been with various antibiotics and shampoos. At the end of the day there didn't seem to be much wrong with him. And yet, as regular as clockwork, Prince Boy's owner, Daisy, a frail looking pensioner in her seventies, would arrive with a list of ailments written down. She also had a knack of picking the busiest of busy days to turn up.

Prince Boy had a cold again. I went over him carefully and found nothing wrong. The dog fixed me with a baleful stare. I got the impression I wasn't the only one who was getting fed up with these constant visits to the vet. I decided that it was time to call her bluff.

'I can't find anything wrong with him, Daisy.'

'Oh,' she answered, a bit taken aback. 'Won't he need an injection and some pills?'

'No. In fact, I'm not going to give him any treatment. We'll just wait and see if anything develops.'

Daisy looked crestfallen. 'Well, could I have some worm pills? I'm sure I saw worms the other day.'

Reluctantly I gave in. Dogs benefit from regular worming so I couldn't see any problem in dispensing a few pills. At least it would reassure Daisy and keep her happy.

The afternoon seemed to go on for ever and I was tired at the end of it. As I left the consulting room I was surprised to see Daisy still in the waiting room, deep in conversation with Mrs Fortuna. She was obviously enjoying herself, if her frequent bursts of laughter were anything to go by. It was a quarter to five. I went back to Prince Boy's clinical record. It showed that Daisy had clocked in at two-fifteen. Even allowing for the long wait, two and a half hours seemed excessive. Then the penny dropped: the hospital had become a home from home for her and she enjoyed the company of the other owners and their pets. The busier the better, for all human life was there! No problem, I thought, but I made a note to warn my colleagues why Prince Boy might not need any treatment on subsequent visits!

The next day was just as hot. I wished it was me on holiday, even though it was only a few weeks since I had been away. Apart from all the flea-related problems making things so busy there was another aspect of the heat which always seems to be a problem in spite of all our attempts to warn people of it. This was an unusual case, though. I was doing the ward rounds and found myself looking at a handsome black cat. She was one of five cats hospitalized for the same thing: they had all fallen great heights from balconies – the dreaded high-rise syndrome. Two of these cats had broken their jaws, one had a split hard palate too. Another had broken both hind legs while the more fortunate of the quartet just had nasty bruising round the face. Those with broken jaws were being fed by the nurses with a tube into the stomach passing through the nose.

I looked at the black cat. She stared back and then, with a little purr, put up her head to be stroked. She had come in during the evening and had been admitted for observation as there didn't seem to be much wrong. I looked at the card. 'Lottie fell 200 feet at 8 p.m. NAD admit obs.' NAD is hospital jargon for 'no abnormality detected'. The vet had signed the card with the time of the examination and the cat had been checked intermittently through the night. She had remained quite normal throughout and now she was ready to go home. I got her out and checked her all over. No pain in the jaw or legs. No evidence of bruising inside the mouth. I had never seen anything like it. We have a lot of experience of high-rise syndrome – unfortunately – and there is no doubt that a lot of avoidable suffering is caused by the carelessness of those owners who live high up with a cat. It is a simple matter to put up a net or restrict access to the danger area in some way.

That day Lottie was sent home with the usual plea not to let it happen again. When I saw a photo of the building she fell from I thought again that her escape was nothing short of a miracle.

Not so lucky was a rabbit who had come in earlier in the hot spell. She had fractured her spine and had had to be put down. Even rabbits are not immune to high-rise syndrome, it seems. For the most part though this is a cat problem, and each year I despair as six to ten patients come in week in week out, in spite of our efforts to warn people of the dangers.

August isn't all doom and gloom, though. Generally speaking, the height of summer is a good time for animals as well as their owners. Dogs get longer walks in the evening sunshine, their owners get more exercise, and infectious illnesses tend to take a back seat, apart from parvo virus, which is ever-present and waiting to strike against unvaccinated puppies allowed out on the streets. One unusual victim of a summer pastime was Shep, a long-haired collie type dog, who was on my operating list on a Tuesday morning in the middle of the month. I had seen him in the clinic the previous afternoon shaking his head violently. His young owners, John and Ruth, both students, had been having a party in their garden on Sunday afternoon and Shep had been quite excited with the general horseplay. Rushing about the garden he had collided with the burning barbecue, dislodged a couple of chops and made off with them. At the time a couple of burning coals had landed on his head. His owners caught him and soaked his head in cold water, which probably was a good thing, especially if there were any hot coals still in his coat. Meanwhile, although Shep had yelped when the charcoal landed on him, he was more interested in his booty than in any pain he might have been feeling.

It wasn't until the next day when John and Ruth surfaced that they noticed Shep was far from well. He was pawing at his head and was obviously in pain, yelping if anyone went near. Placid old dog that he was, there was no way he was going to let me examine his painful head so I had admitted him and given him a pain-killing shot to last him until I could get him under the anaesthetic. We see quite a lot of burns. Coincidentally, we had two cats in ward seven and a rat in ward eight under observation and treatment. They had been rescued by the fire brigade and rushed to us suffering from smoke inhalation as well as burns.

The major worry about burns injuries is that they almost invariably get worse before they improve. Shep was a case in point: although immediately after his accident he had seemed reasonably well, now there was a nasty oozing wound by his ear and on his head. Emma, his nurse for the operation, held him gently under the jaw and brought up his vein so that I could inject the anaesthetic into him, which would allow us to clip the wound and make a thorough examination without causing him distress.

Twenty minutes later the full extent of the damage was visible: two full-thickness burns the size of oranges on his head. Full thickness means that the whole of the outer layer of the skin – the epidermis – has been damaged, which in turn means that healing will take much longer. It is also potentially life-threatening if too much of the body surface has been damaged. Shep's burns were much more extensive than I had thought at first, and there were areas to the side of the main burns that were very red-looking and likely to get worse. He would have to stay in for daily injections of pain-killers, gentle bathing and application of special creams. Worst of all, as far as Shep was concerned, he would have to wear a 'Buster' collar – which looks rather like an Elizabethan ruff – round his neck to prevent him scratching the wounds as they healed. Dogs' eyes are very expressive and poor old Shep looked thoroughly miserable at this latest affront to his dignity. Needs must, though, and I reckoned it would be a couple of weeks before his burns had healed sufficiently for the collar to come off.

A few days later he was fit enough to go home for Ruth and John to tend him. Fortunately, being students, they would be at home most of the time as it was the summer vacation. They turned up to pick him up one afternoon just as a thunderstorm broke. Shep hated storms and, sure enough, as Emma went to get him out of his cage she found him shivering at the back, refusing to come out. Even the familiar presence of his owners didn't seem to pacify him and he tried to climb on to Ruth's lap. There was nothing for it: he would need a sedative to go home with. After a little jab he calmed down just as the torrential rain eased off and he was settled in the back of the car for the ride home. The poor chap had had a trying time of it recently, but at least he would sleep like a log that night.

The downpour had decimated the usual crowds and by four p.m. the waiting room was empty. Empty, that is, except for Prince Boy, who was in again, scratching this time. Daisy hadn't bothered to check at Reception, saying to me that she had been quite happy to wait. With a sigh I looked at her dog. Not a false alarm this time: I caught two fleas. Daisy was delighted – something was definitely wrong – and she skipped out with four months' supply of flea treatment to solve that particular problem and maybe take us up to Christmas. I was certain she'd be in before then, though!

Meanwhile the two cats that had been in the fire were doing well. It was now coming up to a week since they had arrived and their breathing was normal. Quite often, in these cases, complications set in at around the fourth day, usually difficulty in breathing caused by lung congestion. Their owner was still in hospital so it would be a while yet before they could be reunited. Unfortunately the rat hadn't fared so well. He had had quite severe burns around his face and gradually went downhill. He refused food and then developed severe infection in the burned tissue. I had to put him down. Failure to save animals is something every vet has to face up to and you learn to accept this, but I was particularly sad for that little fellow.

It doesn't pay to dwell on failure though, and I prefer to take the optimistic view that it is usually followed up with a successful case. When this is against all the odds it is even sweeter, and on one of the final ward rounds of the month I saw this for myself.

Gabriel was going through a successful run when everything he did went to plan and Sasha, a middle-aged Staffordshire bull terrier, was a triumph. She had grabbed an entire chop bone from the rubbish bin. Attempts to get it out of her mouth had provoked her to swallow it whole. It became apparent that it was going to cause major problems when she vomited her evening meal almost straight after eating it. The same thing happened the next day at breakfast and Sasha's owners suspected that the bone was stuck in her gullet.

When Gabriel heard the story from the owners he admitted Sasha for a chest X-ray: this would show definitively whether or not the bone was stuck in the gullet and exactly where it was. There are three places where bones can get stuck: the entrance to the chest, just above the heart, and just before the stomach. Of these, the most difficult to work on is the area above the heart, which is where Sasha's stolen bone was located. And as Gabriel could see on the X-ray, it was well and truly stuck.

In this situation there are limited options: one is to push the bone down into the stomach using a stomach tube; another is to attach a grasper to the bone using an endoscope and pull it back up through the mouth. Neither of these two options could be considered as either of them would tear the gullet, causing further serious injuries. The only solution, therefore, in Sasha's case would be to open up the chest, locate the bone and cut into the gullet so that it could be removed. This would be a major undertaking and take up the best part of two hours.

The most risky aspect of such operations is the anaesthesia. Elaine, one of the nursing supervisors, had this big responsibility. As soon as Gabriel went into the dog's chest Elaine had to take over her breathing. She did this by pumping the anaesthetic bag connected to the dog's lungs. Gabriel quickly located the bulge in the gullet where the bone was located. A cut into the bulge and out popped the bone. Next the gullet had to be stitched up, which required great care: if the wound broke down subsequently there would be little hope for Sasha. Half an hour later the chest wall had been sewn up and, to everyone's great relief, Sasha had started to breathe on her own. Lastly a chest drain was put in to siphon out any secretions. The operation could not have gone better, and the entire team, plus at the end of the day several of the other nurses, celebrated with a few drinks in the pub across the road.

Sasha was a real survivor and very tough – to look at her a couple of days later you wouldn't have thought that she had been through life-threatening surgery. Yet at this stage a couple of things could still go wrong. The first was wound breakdown, as already mentioned, which would cause infection. This would be a real disaster, and Gabriel tried to avoid this by having the dog on fluids only for three days and by giving full doses of antibiotics. The second problem might occur weeks or months after the operation when scar tissue might cause the gullet to become constricted and make it impossible for the dog to swallow solid food.

133

However, once Sasha had been in for a week, she was taking semi-solid food with gusto so it was time for her to go home.

It was just the sort of triumph on which to end the month. Later that day, I came across the reunion between Sasha and her owners. The dog was jumping all over the place making that wailing sound peculiar to Staffies. Her owners were just as excited and almost in tears with relief that she had made it. This is the stuff that makes it all worthwhile, and even though I hadn't been involved in Sasha's treatment I felt just as happy for her as if I had done all the hard work.

It had been a month of lovely weather, of barbecues, country walks, and the mainly successful treatment of nearly three thousand animals. It would soon be September, my birthday month, and I wondered what dramas would unfold. August had been fulfilling, if slightly chaotic, and I didn't expect much change until the cold weather and shorter days returned – and the fleas retreated.

August concluded on a happy note: the two cats who had been in the fire were pronounced well enough to go home. They were taken by one of the drivers to Phil, their owner, who was also out of hospital now and in temporary accommodation. Apparently he burst into tears when they were brought back to him. I am sure that being together again would mean a more rapid recovery for them all.

SEPTEMBER

The warm weather continued in September with all its attendant problems for our pets. All summer we had managed somehow to get the strays out to homing centres but there are far too many cats for too few owners. It's a constant struggle which in an ideal world we could prevent with neutering and responsible pet ownership. I live in hope!

One good thing was that the BBC cameras were back to film a new series of *Animal Hospital*. By now – after three years – we were welcoming back the production team and camera operators as old friends. Suddenly the hospital was buzzing and even busier. I reckon some people like the idea of being on television and the numbers of patients increase for that reason. It was also good to welcome back Rolf Harris with his tremendous ability to put people at their ease – not to mention his unlimited store of jokes.

The allergy season continued unabated and one case stuck in my memory. This was a Sharpei dog. I rarely see this breed but three turned up within the first week of September. When I qualified I had never heard of them and even ten years ago they were incredibly expensive – which is perhaps why I saw so few as I work in a charity clinic. Nowadays, though, they are easier to come by, so I have begun to see more. Perhaps due to indiscriminate breeding, they have their fair share of problems. Their wrinkled skin predisposes them to infections in its huge folds. They also suffer from demodectic mange, allergies – particularly atopy – and 'cherry eye'.

But my first case of the month was nothing out of the ordinary for September: it was just the scale of it that intrigued me. The eighteen-month-old Sharpei, Shannon, came in late one Sunday afternoon with a swollen nose. The diagnosis was easy: his owner had seen him snapping at several wasps hovering around a tea table in the garden. He had eaten at least two but then had suddenly yelped and retreated into the house pursued by several other angry wasps. For the next hour Shannon seemed subdued and was left alone until one of the children noticed that his face had swollen. Then he was rushed into the hospital. Wasp and bee stings are common in the late summer and aren't usually life-threatening. Nearly always the lips or the nose are affected but the only real danger occurs if the wasp stings after having been eaten: swelling at the back of the throat can cause breathing difficulty.

This is what I was worried about when I first clapped eyes on Shannon's sorry countenance. He was pawing at his face and seemed quite distressed. Before I could get too worried, though, the family told me he was a natural actor and a bit of a wimp. Once on the surgery table he started to play and paw at me, his pain momentarily forgotten. I stood back and watched him. Although he was panting a bit, normal for any dog feeling stressed on the vet's table, there was no evidence of any difficulty in breathing. Then I checked the colour of his lips – nice and pink. Nothing to worry about then: the swelling was just on his face. An injection of pain-killer, in case he wasn't entirely acting, plus another of corticosteroid to reduce the swelling, and we could expect him to be back to normal within twenty-four hours. In 99 per cent of such cases this is what happens; just a few

136

need an additional injection a day or so later.

Another characteristic of Sharpeis is that they have unusual puffy skin: it contains a great deal of a substance called mucin, which thickens the underlying layer, the dermis, and accounts for the puffiness. One little puppy I shan't forget came in a few days later for a second visit. The owners, a nice family, had called her Fat Feet – a really odd name until you saw her paws. I had never seen anything like them. They were *fat*! The puppy was a crossbreed Sharpei but had a lot of the Sharpei in her: she had the distinctive wrinkles – and those fat paws. After going over her for the first time I couldn't find anything to account for the puffiness. I had immediately checked the popliteal lymph nodes at the back of the knee joints: if these were blocked by some disease process, swelling would have resulted, but they were normal. In fact, the swelling didn't seem to bother the pup so my instinct was to leave well alone and see if she grew out of it. She was only four weeks old so we had plenty of time, although decisions would have to be made in about two months if her paws were still abnormal. Specifically we would have to decide whether to put her down if she was unable to walk properly.

I had asked the owner, Jill, to come in again and now she was back with a bigger, bouncier and still funny-looking Fat Feet, who was calm and patient on the examining table, much easier to examine than most puppies. Since her last visit I had been through my books and come up with what I thought was the probable diagnosis: cutaneous mucinosis, which essentially means that the dog has an excessive amount (even for a Sharpei) of mucin in the dermis. There would be no cure for this but, if I was right, it wouldn't get worse and might improve with age. To prove the diagnosis I would have to biopsy the skin and after getting the agreement of Jill and her family I booked Fat Feet in for the next day.

The process of taking a biopsy couldn't be simpler. There was no need for a general anaesthetic. A jab of sedative produced a sleepy puppy and then, under local anaesthetic, I took a small amount of tissue from Fat Feet's leg and sent it to my histopathologist. She's a friend and I can't firmly diagnose certain diseases without her help. Specialists with this kind of expertise hardly existed when I first qualified and, looking back, I wonder how I managed with some unusual ailments. In Fat Feet's case it would be the only way to confirm my diagnosis.

A few days later, I read a report that confirmed my suspicions about Fat Feet's problem. Unfortunately it also confirmed that there was no treatment. I phoned Jill and suggested we leave matters for another month before doing anything. I just kept my fingers crossed that it wouldn't get any worse: putting a pup to sleep is never easy, and Fat Feet had endeared herself to everyone.

My third Sharpei of the month – and of the year – came in the next day with a very different problem, an eye disease with which I was familiar. One look at 'cherry eye' is all it takes to understand its name. Dogs and cats have three eyelids, the third being normally retracted into the corner of the eye. Sometimes the third eyelid of the cat becomes obvious, spreading across the front of the eye, when the cat is run down or suffering from a viral condition. Lining the eyelid, which is also called the nictitating membrane or, in Latin, the *membrana nictitans*, is the Harderian gland. Occasionally this gland gets partially detached from the third eyelid and sticks out in front of the eye like a cherry. This is what had happened to Scrub, a friendly little fellow of only six months old.

At college I had been taught to remove the gland, quite a simple operation and usually effective, but surgical fashions have changed: all the recent graduates starting work at the Harmsworth have told me I should stitch it back in place. I was intrigued to see what my textbooks advised but they described both techniques without much comment. A few weeks before I had found an old textbook on animal eye disease in a second-hand bookshop. It had been written by a French doctor of veterinary surgery, published in 1914 and translated into English. I was amazed to discover an excellent description of the condition, mentioning that it was first described in an Italian dog in 1880. In my book Professor Nicholas recommended stitching the gland back and only removing it if the first operation failed. Which is pretty much what we do now.

I have a small collection of old veterinary books, some of them hundreds of years old, and it is always fascinating to dip into them. Although some were written in the nineteenth century, before the advent of the discoveries that revolutionized all medicine and their authors had no idea of the causes of diseases which we take for granted today, they offered fantastic descriptions of the signs and symptoms, and sometimes the advice on what to do is appropriate today. I learned just as much about cherry eye from my 1914 book as from my modern ones. Another book, at least 150 years old, includes pages and pages on the signs of rabies, which, of course, hasn't been seen in the UK for many decades but which was a common, dreaded sight in the nineteenth century.

Later that day Scrub was given an anaesthetic in the prep room and I stitched the gland back in place which took around ten minutes, although it would be a month or so before I would be able to say whether it had been successful or not. If the answer was yes, I would be grateful to Dr Nicholas, late of Alfort, and who, it seems, had achieved most of his expertise as a major in the French Army at the turn of the century, for his clear description of the disease. I bet he would have been tickled pink if he had been able to foresee that a colleague, and an Englishman at that, could benefit from his experience almost a hundred years later!

A week later it was still incredibly warm, which brought an unwelcome upsurge in balcony cases. A lovely little cat called Lulu had been admitted late at night having apparently 'jumped' into the darkness from a third-floor flat. Usually she went down three flights of stairs and left the building whenever someone came into the block but this had led to her original undoing as she had not been spayed. At eight months she was already expecting kittens. It is not often appreciated that cats (kittens really) as young as four and a half months can come into season and that tom cats are not fussy about the age of the animals they mate with. So there, on my ward rounds, was Lulu in ward seven with a broken shin bone and pelvis. Also she was at least eight weeks pregnant, a week to delivery. She had been X-rayed already, which showed that the shin bone would need a pin inserted. This is a relatively simple operation that involves putting a stainless-steel pin, rather like a knitting needle, right into the centre of the bone through the marrow thus holding the two broken bits together.

The pelvis was a different matter. Most broken-pelvis cases in cats, and we see thousands every year, will heal in six to eight weeks with rest in a cage. Many sufferers have trouble urinating for up to a week and will need constant pain-killers. They are always looked after by the nurses round the clock. I doubted that Lulu would be able to give birth naturally. She sat quite still, looking at me through the bars of her cage, a picture of abject misery, with that pinched look cats have when they are in pain. Thankfully she was able to control her bladder but any movement made her cry out. I increased her pain-killing injections to three times daily. With the pelvic injuries I reckoned a Caesarean section was on the cards and we would have to keep an eye on her over the next few days. Why she had jumped out into the void remained a mystery but we thought she had probably been chasing a fly. Meanwhile, her owners had hung some netting over the balcony window to keep their other cat from a similar fate. Too late to help Lulu.

The next morning, having removed a temporary splint, I fixed Lulu's leg and was pleased to see her back in her cage in the afternoon looking a lot more comfortable, but my pleasure was short-lived. A few hours later she went into labour and was screaming in pain with each contraction. For the second time in a day she had to undergo a major operation. Half an hour later we delivered two live, fairly healthy kittens and Lulu had been spayed. My original estimate that she still had a week to go had been wrong because these two kittens looked as though they had arrived on time. It wasn't ideal with their mother nursing a repaired broken leg, but the next morning, I saw Lulu lying on her side with her bad leg sticking up in the air and two kittens tucking into an ample supply of milk. She was even purring! It was obvious that motherhood had made her forget her fall and her injuries. The worst was over. She would need six weeks of rest to allow the leg to heal then further X-rays would be taken to see when the pin could come out.

It isn't just cats that suffer from being on balconies in warm weather. It's a sad fact that dogs often spend most of their lives stuck on balconies with virtually no exercise. This is mainly because the owners are at work during the day and they don't want the dogs to mess in the flat. Usually they are solitary dogs and to alleviate their boredom they may bark incessantly, causing great nuisance and complaints. The frustrating thing is it's difficult to get evidence of suffering which will stick in a court of law and the only recourse that aggrieved neighbours may have is through the environmental health officer. The sad fact is that unless I can find evidence of disease or physical suffering there won't usually be enough evidence to go to court with. This is a very frustrating state of affairs for all concerned, but not half as frustrating as spending a day in court without a result.

Even though I had come across this problem before, I wasn't prepared for what Inspector Hopgood had been alerted to and brought into the hospital. *Nine* dogs were being kept in a cramped high-rise flat with a balcony. The inspector had been alerted to their predicament by an anonymous phone call. As he brought them out of the flat they seemed confused by being outdoors and the camera crew had to keep well back to avoid alarming them even further.

The nine dogs, all of a small terrier type and probably related to each other, were different from the usual balcony complaint, first in their numbers. I had never had to examine nine dogs in a cruelty case before and each had similar problems. They were all undernourished, between 25 per cent and 50 per cent of proper body weight. When I examined them Rolf Harris was with me, and I demonstrated to him how I could span their abdomens with one hand. They also had overgrown claws. I thought it unlikely that they had ever been out for adequate walks. Most had severe dental problems with gum disease. They all had foul-smelling coats, indicating that they had not been bathed recently – or ever. The conditions they were being kept in were obvi-

142

ously unsatisfactory. All in all it was one of the worst cases of neglect I had seen.

Due to lack of space in the hospital I had all the dogs transferred to private kennels and placed in the care of a private veterinary surgeon with extensive experience of cruelty cases. Over the next few months a great deal of care would be required to get the dogs back to full health and make them into good prospects for new homes after the inevitable court case. Surprisingly after the way they had been treated, they all had lovely natures and would make excellent pets.

They needed blood tests, which showed most of them to be anaemic due to lack of adequate food. Nearly all required general anaesthetics to remove rotten teeth and clean the rest. They had to be treated for worms and fleas and, of course, bathed. I hoped that the severity of the case and the obvious suffering would lead to a substantial ban on the keeping of dogs – for me, this is the satisfying aspect of cruelty-case work. We only take the serious cases to court, but there are many borderline cases which lead to warnings and monitoring. If I had my way, all those found guilty of causing unnecessary suffering would be banned from keeping animals for life.

After the examinations both I and my colleague prepared statements to start the prosecution of the owners, and all the clinical records were put in a safe place to be brought to court when required. We must use only notes taken at the time of the initial examination. An amazing amount of paperwork goes into a prosecution case. Everything has to be done by the book, and quite rightly too or the defending solicitor will make mincemeat of you in the cross-examination. I hoped that the case would come to court quickly so that the dogs could be rehomed.

Towards the middle of the month, back on my ward rounds, I was struggling as usual with large numbers of abandoned cats. One took my fancy, a lumbering, affectionate tom cat. He seemed to love everybody, even the vets who passed his cage. The worst of it was that he could see only through one eye – the other had been injured and was now badly diseased with no hope of saving the sight. We had many more cats than spaces so I had to decide what to do with Nelson. The next day the operating list was horrendous but the nurses reckoned he could be fitted in. He would have to have his eye removed and the sooner the better. We could anticipate healing within ten days when he would be ready for rehoming if his owner had not come forward. Curiously, one-eyed cats (who nearly always seem to be rechristened Nelson) are generally easy to find homes for. The sight of a friendly and usually a tom cat with one eye seems to bring out the strongest caring emotions in prospective owners.

The next day Stan operated on Nelson, and half an hour later he was coming round, purring in his sleep as though he knew better times were just round the corner. Eye enucleation, as it is called, is not a difficult operation. First we sew the eyelids together, then carefully dissect out the eye. It is not for the squeamish, as you might imagine, and it is not an operation that I enjoy, but it is the only thing we can do for badly damaged or diseased eyes. I reckoned Nelson had lost his eye fighting and, judging by the neglected state of him, I just couldn't imagine that he had a caring owner, which was all the more curious when you considered his love of all humans – he really was an exceptionally friendly cat. At the end of his operation he was castrated, which would put an end to his fighting days, and vaccinated – everything in fact that would make him homeable. We also tested him for the feline Aids virus, which is much more common in male cats, being transmitted in saliva via bite wounds. The test was negative, thank goodness.

The reports nurse, meanwhile, had been her usual industrious self, phoning all our contacts throughout the south-east in the daily effort to shift the strays. Less than 10 per cent are ever claimed so it's a never-ending but important task to place them. There was jubilation when Jackie got Nelson into the Mayhew home in north-west London. This remarkable place rescues and rehomes thousands of cats each year and is a great boon to us at the Harmsworth. Even better, Nelson could go tomorrow as their trained staff would be well qualified to nurse him and take out his stitches.

The next day I was at the Mayhew: one of the Harmsworth vets goes there every morning to neuter animals for anyone in the local area unable to afford a private vet's fees. Half-way through the session, I noticed a young couple with two children pass the operating theatre on their way to the cattery. I was told they wanted to replace their much-loved cat that had recently died of old age. A thought ran through my head: What about Nelson? It was as though my thoughts had been read, because ten minutes later Helen, one of the staff, popped her head round the door and said, 'Can you tell me anything about the cat that has had his eye out?' I gave her all the information I could, adding what a lovely cat he was and that he deserved a break and anything else I could think of! A few minutes later she was back: Nelson was reserved, pending a home check on the couple! I was delighted.

The home check would be a formality, I was sure. It's RSPCA policy to be careful that animals are homed in good circumstances and we do this through home checks. It's a little time-consuming but it benefits the cat, who can be guaranteed a far better life than he has ever known before. The young couple lived in a quiet suburb with a huge garden and the wife was at home all day, having taken time out to bring up her family. As the family were passing I asked them why they had decided to take Nelson out of the hundred or so other cats needing homes. Apparently he had purred like mad as soon as one of the young daughters stroked him and he had rolled over on his back to have his tummy tickled. With his one eye they had simply fallen for him. I couldn't wait to get back to the Harmsworth and tell the nurses who had looked after him. It was Friday and would make the week for them.

Towards the middle of the month an old tom cat called Tiggy was brought into the morning clinic. The previous day Jeremy had seen him with an amazing number of ticks stuck to his face and head. There were others elsewhere on his body but the majority seemed to have accumulated round his head – so many that he could hardly see. Removing ticks is really a job for an expert. The worst thing to do is to try to pick them off because it's the easiest thing in the world to leave the head in. The cat's immune system regards this as a 'foreign body' and then mounts a response that results in an inflamed area which the cat scratches, causing infection. Many suggestions have been made over the years as to the best way to kill the ticks prior to removing them, ranging from a cigarette lighter under the tick (a *very* bad idea!) to solvents like acetone. We like to spray them with special insecticide, then wait until they are dead before carefully removing them. Jeremy had sprayed each tick with a little squirt of insecticide and asked the owner to come back in the morning. Hopefully the creatures would be dead and the risk of leaving their heads in the cat would be much reduced.

Poor Tiggy looked a sight with at least twenty ticks stuck fast on his face and neck. Getting them off took half an hour. After experimenting with various types of forceps I finally found that it was easiest to use my finger and thumb and prise them off. They were pretty tough ticks, too, because I soon found that they were still alive. Tiggy's owner, Sid, an old gentleman living on his own, suddenly said, ''Ere, that one's moving!'

I had carefully teased one tick after another off the cat's face, put them on the consulting table and had taken no notice of them while concentrating on the next. Sure enough, not one but several ticks were scuttling across the table. Suddenly Sid didn't look well. 'Blimey, I feel sick,' he said. Ticks have that effect on some people and the sight of several seedy-looking ones ambling silently across the table was too much for poor old Sid. He had to leave the room and sit down. Meanwhile, Tiggy was taking it in his stride and even, incredibly, purring – although, come to think of it, having several ticks removed from your face must be a relief! When I was sure that I had removed them all, the cat was given a final spray of insecticide. The ticks had probably survived the first attack because it was difficult to spray enough on the face, given the proximity of the eyes, to kill them. It had been enough to make them sickly, though, and easier to remove than would have been the case otherwise.

I was intrigued to see if I could identify what species they were. Relatively few ticks are known to attack dogs and cats in the UK and after consulting my parasitology book I was fairly certain that they were *Ixodes hexagonus*, the tick normally found on hedgehogs, although they will hop on to dogs and cats. Ticks have an interesting life-cycle because at each developmental stage, larva, nymph and adult, they have to find a host, feed on blood, then drop off before developing into the next stage. They often turn out to be three-host ticks. Sid lived in a basement flat with access to a garden and loved to leave out food for 'his' hedgehogs. No doubt Tiggy and the hedgehogs had shared a resting place, which was how Tiggy had come to be infested, although it was a mystery to me why his face had been so badly attacked. As I was looking down the microscope at the mouth parts of one of the ticks I had just prised off I couldn't help but wonder at the intricacy of the little creature. Unlike Sid, I was enjoying myself.

Meanwhile, in the skin clinic, I was getting somewhere near a diagnosis with a yellow Labrador that had been intriguing me for several months. Teddy was two years old and had been scratching for almost a year. He had come in during February with a few fleas but flea control hadn't helped a great deal. A short burst of steroids stopped the scratching but as soon as the pills were finished, back came the itching. It had all the hallmarks of an allergy – but to what?

Teddy's owner, Bill, agreed to help us with an allergy investigation. First, food. Food allergy is a controversial subject among vets: some think it's very common and others it's very rare. Whatever the truth, though, you certainly won't diagnose it without looking for it! This involves putting the dog on a diet that, as far as anyone is aware, he has never eaten before. In Teddy's case, this consisted of rabbit, rice and water – nothing else. It would have to be given for at least six weeks and possibly a month longer than that. The theory is that once the allergic component of the diet has been eliminated from the system and continues to be excluded the dog's itchiness will disappear. The next step would be to go back to the original diet: if food allergy exists, back would come the itching within a few days.

Now Teddy sat in front of me scratching his ears and tummy. He had been on the diet for seven weeks and was not at all improved. There was no point in continuing along this track. Bill stared sadly at his dog. I could sense his frustration, especially after the mammoth task of cooking rabbit and rice daily for nearly two months. Reading his thoughts, I said, 'Well, I don't think it's been a waste of time, Bill. At least we know he isn't allergic to fleas or food.'

When I encouraged him Teddy obligingly jumped up on the table. Like many Labradors he would willingly participate in the examination as though it were a game. I looked at his mouth, ears, armpits and tummy. For this part he rolled over with all four legs in the air. He had itchy red ears, and a very inflamed tummy. Also, the back of his paws were reddened from his constant licking. It looked more than ever like the allergic disease called atopy, which is similar to asthma or hay fever in people. In dogs and cats the disease is a skin problem, and over the last few months Teddy had developed more of the typical signs as I had ruled out other allergies.

I explained all this to Bill and suggested that as Teddy was such a young dog it might be worth doing an allergy test to see if we could identify the cause of the allergy and if he agreed I intended to do it that afternoon. It is nice to know exactly what a dog (or cat) is allergic to but often it doesn't change the treatment. It's a bit like knowing exactly what pollens cause your hay fever – interesting, but you are still going to depend on antihistamines or nasal sprays to control symptoms. Skin tests are potentially useful, however, if we want to try a vaccine against the allergy, but even then there is no guarantee that it will work, and it might take up to nine months before we know if it has been successful. It was a long shot but because Teddy was so young I thought it was worth it.

Later that day, he lay on the operating table heavily sedated. We have to sedate dogs like Teddy because many injections are given in allergy skin tests – up to fifty is possible. After the first half dozen or so even the most phlegmatic dog, like Teddy, is apt to get upset. I injected forty possible allergens – substances to which Teddy might be allergic – into his skin and fifteen minutes later I examined each injection site. When the reaction is positive, a red bump appears almost immediately. Teddy had lots of angry-looking red bumps. He was allergic to different pollens, some moulds and, like many other dogs, to house-dust mite.

We decided to attack on several fronts. First a vaccine, supplemented with high doses of evening-primrose oil, antihistamines, special shampoos and plenty of vacuuming to try to reduce the house-dust mite. Finally Teddy would be banned from his owner's bedroom as this is the place where most dust accumulates. One thing was certain: I was going to see a lot of this dog over the next six months. I watched him wagging his tail and gazing up at his master while we talked about him and felt determined to improve his quality of life. Being constantly itchy can't be much fun and he was only two.

With winter beckoning and colder weather not far off I felt this was as good a time as any to get Teddy under better control. Most of the pollens to which he was allergic would be gone for the time being, leaving the moulds and house-dust mite as the main enemies. However, as I glanced out of my office window on one of the last days of September it

150

was difficult to believe that summer was supposed to be more or less over. It was a lovely day with a shimmering heat haze, like the best of August, and not a cloud in the sky. There was a lovely atmosphere in the hospital with most of the nurses having had time off and looking tanned and healthy. Lunch times were spent sitting outside in the court-yard at the back. A few lucky ones had chosen to take this week off and were in Cornwall, basking in sunshine more typical of Spain. For poor old Teddy, though, the prolonged heat just made his itchiness worse. He would have to have a cold shower out in the garden tonight before going to bed in the kitchen.

On the last day of September I found myself confronted with Joe, an exuberant Staffordshire bull terrier. Of course, this breed is naturally exuberant, but in Joe's case it went beyond what anyone could call reasonable. He was in my clinic for a tummy upset but it was quickly apparent that this was not the real issue. His attack of diarrhoea and sick-ness had started two days ago and was getting better. His owner, Jeannie, had brought him in for a check-up. This soon established that there wasn't much wrong with him physically. At eighteen months old, you could perhaps describe him as a teenager in dog terms. Getting him on to the table took half a dozen attempts. He was on the table and off the other side (twice), ran round the room (twice), and after that just rolled over and played dead when I tried to pick him up. That's quite difficult with a dead weight and he was big for a Staffie. Then, just as I thought I'd cracked it, he jumped out of my arms. There was no maliciousness – he did all this with yelps and frantic wagging of his tail, and the high-pitched wail which sounds almost human and which any vet familiar with the breed will recognize as typical Staffie.

'He's a bit manic, if you don't mind me saying so!' I puffed when at last he was ready for the examination.

Later, the whole story came out. Manic was the word. Joe never seemed to rest and the real reason for the consultation wasn't the tummy upset, it was the strain of living with Joe, not only for Jeannie but her entire family. This is a scenario often seen by vets. The actual reason for the consultation is not immediately apparent in some cases. A lot of people are embarrassed to admit that their pet, which they love, is nonetheless a bit of a pain to live with. Or in Joe's case, more than a bit of a pain. How can you broach the subject with the vet? To say that the dog is intolerable to live with doesn't seem to be something 'to waste a vet's time with'. And in any case, what can one realistically expect a vet to be able to do in such a situation? The answer is quite a lot these days.

But first I had to establish that Joe was indeed bringing the family to their knees and why. He had been a rescue dog – we were beginning to see why – and there was no indication of how he had been treated in his early days. Jeannie was the third owner in his short life and she had had him for three months. The ideal time to acquire a dog to make training easiest is just after weaning at eight weeks. This is the time when the foundations for a good relationship with humans are built. Lots of love at this stage plus security and knowing the boundaries of what is acceptable sets up good behaviour of the sort we all want from man's best friend. I suppose it's roughly comparable to the first four years of a child's life. By the time the dog is four or five months old, patterns may have been set that are difficult to change later on. I have seen so many dogs that have had no training as pups. Some owners leave them in flats all day then punish them if they have soiled the home. Pretty soon the pup learns to fear the turning of the key in the lock, expecting a beating. The owner will then say, 'He always looks guilty when he's been bad.' Other puppies are acquired at four to five months without much socialization either with humans or other animals and straight away are at a disadvantage. Some veterinary surgeries now run puppy socialization classes to get round this problem. Apart from the obvious advantage to the owner, a well-adjusted dog is more pleasant to treat in later years!

Who knows what sort of life Joe had had in his first six crucial months of life? Likely as not, he had been left for long periods. He clearly craved human attention, as if he was scared stiff of being left again. He was always wanting to play, always initiating the interactions with Jeannie. She told me that he couldn't be left without trashing the room he was in – so much so that whenever he had to be alone the bathroom was chosen. Even this room was now in urgent need of redecorating and a new door would have to be ordered. When he wasn't making a mess he would bark and howl, which had brought complaints from the neighbours. On Jeannie's return home he would urinate submissively. Friends had started to make excuses not to visit since Joe constantly pestered them by jumping up and whining or pawing them for attention. He was a continual attention-seeker and simple pleasures like sitting in front of a favourite television programme had ceased to exist. Even outside it was no better. He would pull incessantly on the lead, and when released he would dash off and refuse to come when called. If he was left off the lead, a short walk might last a couple of hours while Jeannie tried to catch up with him. On one occasion she had given up and gone home. Three hours later Joe had turned up covered in mud.

Sorting Joe out and turning him into an acceptable

companion was going to be difficult. The biggest problem in situations like this is time – which most vets don't have enough of. I decided to phone a few contacts who might be able to help. In spite of all the trials and tribulations it was plain that Jeannie loved her dog and didn't want to get rid of him. A fourth owner would not be easy to find and, unless something could be done, Jeannie was destined for a life of being ruled by her pet! However, it seemed to me that much of Joe's behaviour was predictable for a dog, albeit over the top, and what he needed was a consistently applied training programme to put Jeannie back in the driving seat as the boss. As I started to phone round I reckoned that it might be a few months before any benefit would start to show. I pencilled in a repeat consultation for November so I could see how things were going.

Nowadays there are quite a few pet behaviour specialists and some of these are veterinary surgeons too. Ten years ago few of us knew much about behavioural problems in pets or where to send the owners of such animals for help. But we now know that results are excellent as long as the owner is dedicated and patient. Looking at Jeannie as I fixed up an appointment I was optimistic.

OCTOBER

Over the years I've got very used to the cameras – perhaps too used to them as now I find myself forgetting that I'm being watched by millions of viewers. Early in the month I had my first chance in this series to look really silly. A five-year-old Yorkshire terrier called Bill was brought in by his owner, a widowed pensioner whose son had given her the dog when her husband had died. The two of them had been inseparable since. But over the last month or so a rather horrible smell had become noticeable around Bill. All Elsie knew was that friends were complaining to her and visiting less frequently!

Foul smells in dogs generally come from the mouth (usually bad breath), ears, sometimes from skin disease, and therefore from the coat, or from the area around the bottom and most often associated with two little sacs called the anal sacs or glands. We put Bill on the table, where he stood patiently, and started at the front. I leaned close and smelt his ears and mouth. Elsie followed suit. Everything seemed normal. Next I looked at his teeth but these were strong and clean so no obvious problem there. His coat seemed fine too. I had a good smell, as did Elsie. Being a dog, Bill seemed to accept all this sniffing as normal. I drew the line at the anal sacs.

These are to be found just inside the anus at four o'clock and eight o'clock and cause no end of problems. They don't have any function in modern, domesticated dogs but in the wild they almost certainly serve as a means for dogs to advertise their presence and stake out territory. As the dog passes a motion it squeezes a little of the contents of the sacs over the droppings. Other dogs sniff and find out who's around. The sacs often get blocked and the dog tries to relieve this by scooting along the ground. Sometimes it develops an abscess, which is very painful and needs lancing followed by antibiotics. Very often, as in Bill's case, they cause a foul smell, which might be attractive to dogs but certainly isn't to humans!

I put on some gloves and squeezed out the contents on to some cotton wool. Waving it as near as I dared to Elsie's nostrils I said, 'What about this?' A second or two later I had my answer: Elsie screwed up her face into an expression of such disgust that no one could doubt the diagnosis. I didn't bother to check it myself.

'Has he been scooting along on his bottom?' I asked.

'Well, now you mention it he's been doing that for the last three weeks. I thought he had worms so I gave him some pills I bought in the pet shop,' replied Elsie.

Emptying anal sacs is something vets who treat dogs probably do every day of their working lives. I've often wondered how they come to be called glands as, strictly speaking, a gland is an organ that produces a hormone while the anal sacs produce only a secretion – which, frankly, stinks. Cats have them too but they don't cause anywhere near as many problems. In other animals, such as the skunk, they have developed into a method of self-defence as few creatures can stand the smell. Bill would need his sacs emptying whenever he showed the symptoms, and to help in the immediate future I suggested a bath in some nice-smelling shampoo. Elsie left with a relieved smile – no doubt looking forward to getting back to a more active social life. As for Bill, he had tried to nip

156

me when I squeezed his bottom – no thanks there!

My next case was a gerbil. These are friendly little rodents that make good children's pets. I was interested to read in one of my books recently that they were only introduced into the UK in 1964. Most of the ones we see are Mongolian gerbils, native to Mongolia and north-eastern China. They live for twenty-four to thirty-six months on average, so at twenty months Cheeky was getting on a bit. Like most gerbils he didn't seem to mind me handling him – they rarely bite, which endears them to me. His owner, Tracy, who was four and a half, as she proudly told me, had come in with her mother. It was the first trip to the vet for both of them (and also for Cheeky) so Tracy was just a bit apprehensive.

As soon as you turned him over Cheeky's problem was obvious. There was a large hard swelling on his tummy and in the last few days he had started to nibble at it. This is a well-recognized symptom and there is only one solution. Gerbils have a so-called 'scent gland' which they rub against objects in the wild and to make their presence known. Only other gerbils can detect it – they are probably the cleanest of all the rodents and have no appreciable smell, at least to humans. Occasionally, in older gerbils, the gland develops into a cancer, which without treatment will, like all cancers, keep on growing and therefore has to be removed. Surgery on gerbils is not without risk due to their small size: a few drops of gerbil blood is the equivalent of several pints in a human. One good thing is that the new anaesthetic gases now available have reduced the risk of surgery to these little creatures.

I found myself explaining to a tearful Tracy that her pet would have to have the lump removed or he would suffer and ultimately have to be put down. Of course, she wanted to know if he would die under the anaesthetic and that's a tough one to answer to anyone, but more so with someone so young. 'We'll do our best not to let that happen,' I said, and arranged to have her pet put on that afternoon's list. Cheeky was taken into the hospital and I felt sorry for his owners as they left hand in hand. I noticed that they lived quite close by and just as they were leaving I told them to come back at four rather than ring in. On busy days like today it can take some time to get through and I thought that would be too much for young Tracy.

As it happened the operation was a textbook case. It was done by Bairbre and didn't result in any significant blood loss. Cheeky didn't seem to mind the anaesthetic gas being pumped into a small plastic chamber and he quickly went to sleep. After that he was transferred on to a tiny mask and Bairbre got to work.

It is astounding how quickly the small pets come round from the new gas, within a minute or so of the operation being completed, and at four Tracy and her mum were viewing Cheeky sitting up in his cage seemingly none the worse for his ordeal. They wanted to take him home there and then, but Bairbre thought it best to keep him in, in case he started to interfere with the stitches. In all probability he would go home in the morning, and a happy Tracy skipped out to go home for tea – a complete contrast to the dejected little girl of earlier!

Sure enough, on ward rounds the next day Cheeky seemed quite himself again. I can never get over animals' ability to recover from major surgery – and the smaller they are the tougher they seem to be. Experience has shown us that gerbils are indeed tough little characters.

On the other hand, experience also tells us when an animal has little chance of surviving and we can adapt accordingly. In the same ward as Cheeky was a young hedgehog. We get a lot of them in the hospital all year round. They are known as the gardener's friend and I'm always heartened by the care and attention people lavish on 'their' hedgehogs. They are fascinating creatures, weighing in at 800 to 1200 grams. Pet hedgehogs relying on humans for sustenance can live an amazing ten years but in the wild four is more normal.

Most hedgehogs are born in April or May and are usually independent of Mum by six weeks old, by which time they weigh about 230 grams. Once they get into the slugs they grow quickly. The problem we see in October relates to litters born in September: these young hedgehogs may not survive the winter. Hibernation will occur naturally if the temperature gets below 10 degrees Centigrade but research done in the eighties showed that late-litter hedgehogs that weighed less than 450 grams had virtually no chance of survival. The young hedgehog in the next cage to Cheeky weighed 250 grams but seemed well. The reports nurse would try to place him in a wildlife sanctuary where he could spend the winter in safety without hibernating. Contrary to popular belief, hedgehogs don't have to hibernate, provided they are warm and well fed, and in the wild they probably hibernate intermittently when the temperature is low enough.

A day or so later I was presented with a patient with which I couldn't find anything wrong. This is always baffling and a worry because you think you're missing something, especially when it's a rat, since there isn't a great deal written about them, and even more so when the rat's owner is about to qualify as a doctor. It was midway through the consultation when I realized that this rat's owner knew more than the average person about medical

159

matters. For one thing she was using terms like dyspnoeic, meaning he had a breathing difficulty, and had been slightly anorexic, or not eating.

I came straight out with it. 'Are you medically qualified?'

'Not yet,' replied the young woman, 'but I hope to be next year. I'm in my final year at medical school.' I was quite sure she could do without the extra worry over Boris in addition to the hassle and hard work that final year medical – and veterinary – students face. Jean had had Boris for a couple of years and he travelled everywhere with her. It was touching to see how much she loved him and it seemed to be reciprocated as he wriggled around her neck and up and down her sleeve. He was very much at home!

According to Jean, Boris had apparently been eating a lot better recently but she was still worried. Medical students and doctors are trained to be observant and I had learned over the years to take their worries seriously. Although vets and doctors receive similar training in medical principles I have also found that doctors know little about animal disease just as I know little of human disease. I must admit that with two young children, though, I am learning huge amounts about their ailments and bother our doctor a lot less now than in the early stages! Still, a medical student with a sick rat presented a challenge.

I went over Boris carefully. With a normal temperature and looking bright and inquisitive, he certainly didn't seem ill. His heart was racing nineteen to the dozen but a rat's normal heart-rate is between 300 and 450 beats per minute – an amazing statistic in itself. I could hear absolutely nothing wrong with his chest.

'But don't you think he's breathing a bit fast?' said Jean. I looked up the normal breathing rate of rats. We were both surprised to find out that it was between 70 and 150 breaths per minute. Jean was less worried. And my decision was to do nothing or, as I often call it, 'scientific neglect'. This means that if I can't find anything wrong I don't give any treatment for a few days but ask the owner to keep an eye on things. If there were to be a deterioration I could always do blood tests and X-rays. We were taught at college that we should use sophisticated tests to confirm our clinical suspicions rather than for the sake of it. Jean was happy with this – apparently medical students are told the same thing, which I can understand as multiple tests can be hugely expensive.

The only thing I picked up on was that Boris seemed to prefer hamster food. My rat book advised against this because it contains sunflower seeds and peanuts, which are too high in oils and proteins. It would have to be rat food from now on. That shouldn't be a problem, as rats are well known for their ability to eat just about anything. Boris burrowed into Jean's pullover and they departed, Jean looking a lot happier than when she had come in. I was glad when she rang a few days later and told me I was right – Boris was showing no signs of ill health.

The last case of the day turned out to be more complicated than I would have expected at first sight. Jess, a beautiful ginger and white cat, had come home with what looked like a bit of string sticking out of her mouth. Her owner, Trudy, had given it a tug but it seemed firmly stuck and pulling it upset Jess. I wondered what it would turn out to be. The worst scenario would be cotton thread since a needle might be attached to the end and if that was in the stomach then the cat would be in for major surgery. I opened Jess's mouth as gently as I could and was relieved to see that the thread, or whatever it was, was attached to the carnassial tooth in the upper jaw. This is one of the biggest teeth that dogs and cats have, with three large roots. I did a gentle tug. No joy, it was well and truly anchored.

There was really no choice. Jess would need a general anaesthetic right away because I couldn't leave her pawing at her mouth all night. She was given her premed injection and five minutes later a little anaesthetic into the vein – just enough to knock her out for five minutes, which is all I thought I would need. Now I could really see what was going on. The 'thread' was a stringy piece of grass which had wedged itself tightly between the carnassial tooth and the one next to it. It was as though the cat had been trying to floss her teeth. No wonder it was tight and wouldn't come when pulled. I had to cut it from both ends and then pick the rest out with a fine needle. It took the whole five minutes and Jess was blinking at me as I finished. Half an hour later she would be ready to go home.

As I drove home, later than usual, I reflected on whether I had ever seen a blade of grass stuck in the teeth before. It has often been said that cats and dogs eat grass because of a tummy upset. I reckon it's because they like the taste – and I have seen blades of grass in the back of the throat, up the nose, in the eye but never stuck in the teeth. It was a nice end to the day to have been able to sort it out so quickly.

The next day Fat Feet was back for a check-up. She was now three months old and at crunch time, I suspected, in terms of her outlook. I was a little apprehensive for Jill when I called out her name but I needn't have worried. The broad smiles on her face told me all I needed to know before I had even started questioning. This is so often the case with the frustrating illnesses, with triumphs and failures all mirrored by the owners who can't hide their feelings. Fat Feet was doing well. It seemed that she was growing into her peculiar problem. The fleshy folds were still evident round the joints on her legs but nowhere near as bad, and she was walking quite well. The puffiness was also less marked. I was so pleased and Jill had by now well and truly bonded with her. Fat Feet would be staying put in a good home. It was lovely to be able to say that, unless Jill was worried about anything, I couldn't see the need to bring Fat Feet back to the hospital. I was quite sorry to see them leave – I had got quite attached to Fat Feet myself. She was one of those patients that stand out because they teach you something new.

Just in case I was getting too confident, my next case didn't go to plan. Bill was back in with Teddy and his face told me that things were not progressing. To illustrate his master's worries, Teddy put in a frantic, prolonged spell of scratching all along his tummy and seemed oblivious of our shouting at him to stop. The vaccine was having no effect yet – in fact, poor Teddy was worse. Turning him over and looking at his tummy I had a good idea why: he had a measles-like rash all over, a sign of infection, which was making the original allergy even more itchy. I was disappointed but not surprised – this is a well-known complication with allergies and Teddy would have to go on to high doses of antibiotics for the next month. All was not lost but I could see that Bill needed some encouraging words. Dermatology is a succession of triumphs and failures, and you need patience: most skin diseases take time to control. Teddy was going to need lots of this. The setback made me even more determined to get him better. Armed with a month's supply of potent antibiotics, which I knew to be effective in skin infections, along with antihistamines, evening-primrose oil and vaccines, Bill trudged out. If we weren't seeing improvement in a month, things would be desperate. I didn't even want to think about it. I shut out all thoughts of failure and left that particular worry to November.

Some skin infections are a lot easier to get under control than Teddy's but can be more disastrous in their consequences for the owner. Bruno was a case in point. A beautiful flat-coated retriever, he was only a year old, and full of the joys of spring, which was part of the problem. He was so exuberant that he would bound puppy-like round the house colliding with furniture and knocking things over. His owners could just about cope with all this: Bruno had been a present from their son who thought that his dad, in particular, needed some exercise now that he was retired. And, indeed, he got plenty of that, walking such an active dog for a couple of hours each day.

The problem was that Bruno had developed a chin infection, which made his habit of knocking into things particularly troublesome. Mrs Robinson would continually find pus and blood smeared on the furniture. Something had to be done about it.

Getting a look at Bruno's chin was not easy. There wasn't an ounce of viciousness in him – but he would wriggle and jerk away so that trying to have a proper look was frustrating. After a few minutes' wrestling with him, I had seen enough, though. Bruno had acne – or, at least, its canine equivalent. Canine acne is similar in many ways to the human condition. In dogs it affects the face, but more especially the chin, and usually occurs when the dog is an adolescent of between one and two years of age. Most grow out of it, just like teenagers, but a few are unlucky enough to suffer from the disease for the rest of their lives and in them we can only offer control measures.

Bruno was given a jab of sedative to make further investigation easier. Ten minutes later he was flopped out on the consulting table with great droopy eyes and occasionally deep sighs. The owners could hardly believe their eyes – he was only like this when he was asleep! I did a skin scraping to make sure there weren't any mites and sent a sample of pus to a laboratory to see what germs were causing the problem and, more importantly, to find out what antibiotics would be effective. The infection was quite deep and I thought it might take six weeks or longer to get it under control. The outlook for Bruno was good and I thought that by Christmas we would need to adopt a strategy to prevent the infection coming back. Hopefully by the time he turned two he would grow out of the problem – for his sake and the furniture!

Bruno, although temporarily a bit trying, at least had a loving home. The dog that sticks out in my mind – and probably in the minds of most of our viewers – as one of the most neglected dogs I have seen during the year was Heidi. She had been given the name by Phil, who found her roaming the streets of north-west London. Just about recognizable as a greyhound, she was covered in sores from head to foot. As she wandered about aimlessly, sniffing in dustbins, she had been undoubtedly on her last legs. Phil, who managed to get her on a lead, brought her straight in to us.

I always feel sorry for greyhounds. Enormous numbers are abandoned and, for some reason I have never understood, they are difficult to home. Anyone who has ever owned one will tell you that they are the most gentle of dogs and make excellent pets.

In spite of Heidi's appalling condition her lovely temperament shone through. It didn't matter what I did to her, there was absolute trust and she was calm and gentle – even though she was less than a year old. She raised her head to be petted, shutting her eyes as she did so – the typical gesture of the loving family pet. I hoped we could cure her so that she could become just that.

As soon as we had assessed Heidi we were able to establish what was wrong with her. I did a skin scraping and found demodex mites by the hundred. This parasite is transmitted from the mother to her pups in the first few days of their lives. Many dogs will grow up to be carriers but others, like Heidi, will develop a severe, generalized disease, which can be fatal. In Heidi's case she was not far from the terminal phase. To say she was miserable would be the understatement of the year. Festering sores everywhere on her body meant that she was very itchy, but far too sore to scratch. She had become unwell and refused food.

Phil was adamant that he wanted to give her a home. I felt I had to put him totally in the picture. 'She'll need months of treatment. There will be setbacks and new problems. She will need weekly baths, daily antibiotics and very careful nursing. At the end of all that we might fail – I'd say that was a 50 per cent possibility right now. And if we do she'll have to be put down.'

Phil thought about this for a moment. 'I think she needs a chance. I want to give that to her. She deserves it.' He was close to tears. I am sure Rolf was too as he listened to this conversation and looked down at the poor dog sitting patiently on the table.

So that was it. We would give it our best shot. Heidi would remain with us for a week to try to get her through the critical phase. In addition to bathing with special shampoo she would also have twice-daily injections of potent antibiotics and much cuddling and tempting to eat. We soon discovered that Heidi was a fighter – within a few days she had started to respond. By hand-feeding her, Clare got her to eat some boiled chicken and soon she was gradually getting her appetite back. The bathing process was slow and gentle because the affected skin was so painful, but after a week she was out of immediate danger and the first signs of improvement were beginning to show. The angry redness of her skin had started to fade and we could stroke her without her crying out.

The disease caused by the demodex mite is one of the more difficult skin conditions to cure. It's called demodicosis, or demodectic mange, and has been known since antiquity. In the oldest books, written in medieval times, it was called 'redde mange' and over the years just about everything has been claimed to cure it. Today there is only one product on the market, a shampoo, which has a licence for its treatment. Using this shampoo, along with antibiotics, we have a success rate of over 90 per cent when we start with cases a lot less advanced than Heidi's. One of the main problems is that the mite depresses the immune system and the dogs become susceptible to all sorts of infections of which the most common is a deep pus-filled infection of the skin. This was what Heidi had. It meant that, in addition to weekly baths, she would need months of antibiotics and even though she had improved she was not entirely out of danger.

The next day Phil had a lesson in how to bath dogs with demodectic mange. Clare went through the procedure step by step, making sure that he knew how to dilute the shampoo and then to apply it absolutely everywhere, even on the sore bits which, of course, is the hardest part. Thorough baths would be crucial to the success or failure of the treatment. Looking back over the years on my failures, they had often been due to the inability of the owner to keep up the difficult and often tedious procedures, maybe with setbacks and only near-imperceptible progress. Yet when things go right there are few more satisfying conditions to treat.

I reflected on one very advanced case I had seen some years ago as I watched Phil and Heidi leave the hospital together a week later. Bob Downes was out walking his German shepherd dog in the local park one cold Sunday morning in winter when the dog darted into a bush and came out with something tucked into her mouth. She deposited the object at Bob's feet. At first Bob thought it was just a bundle of rags but when it moved he realized it was alive – but only just. It was a puppy, dying of the cold, shivering and hardly able to stand. Worse, he had lost most of his hair. Bob picked him up and brought him straight round to the hospital. The duty nurse, Jill, admitted the puppy for assessment and, most importantly, warmth and food. It was hard to say, with all that hair loss, but I reckoned that he was probably a Jack Russell of about four months. When he had warmed up and, amazingly, tucked into a plate of food, I looked him over. What remained of his coat was very scaly and the skin underneath had a peculiar slate-blue colour, which immediately made me suspect demodectic mange, but unlike Heidi, the puppy didn't have a skin infection on top. Ten minutes later, thanks to a skin scraping, the diagnosis was confirmed.

Fortunately for the pup, Bob had decided that he wanted to adopt Scrap, as he became known. Sally, his German shepherd, seemed keen too – she had tried to lick and mother him from the moment she rescued him. But, just as in Heidi's case, Bob had to learn that curing dogs involves a huge investment in time and perseverance. Jill took an interest too – in fact, I thought she wanted the pup for herself as she was always around when Bob came in, at first weekly then monthly, for check-ups.

Scrap came on in leaps and bounds. Just four months later almost all his hair had grown back and he was a bouncy, full-of-life Jack Russell again. Bob, of course, was delighted and also amused at how the dog had taken over the household and, in particular, Sally. He would jump up and grab her ear in a friendly way, and the pair would roll about the carpet in mock fights, which Sally always allowed Scrap to win. On the final check-up there was a tear in Jill's eye: we knew that, in all probability, we wouldn't need to see Scrap again, and that was how things turned out.

With those memories in my mind I watched Heidi hop into Phil's car. Dogs take so quickly to kindness in a new owner no matter how badly they have been treated, and I was glad to see that she was confident enough to stick her head out of the window, sniffing the air and apparently revelling in her new freedom as she was driven away. I noticed she had already claimed the front seat next to Phil!

Finding homes for animals is not something I do very much. Thousands of cats, dogs, rabbits and others are homed by the RSPCA every year and it is a full-time job in itself. Each person wanting to adopt a pet has to be checked so that we can be sure the animal is going to the best possible home. It seems only reasonable when you consider that many of those pets have had a bad start in life. I generally leave animal-homing to our centres who specialize in this. There have been exceptions, though, and I found myself having to make hard decisions about a dog called Muffin for whom I found two homes in her long life. Years ago, when I was in private practice, one of my clients had lost her dog and was bereft. She agonized about getting another one but was worried that she wouldn't live long enough to be able to care for it. I thought she was so active that she should get another dog and I finally persuaded her by addressing her main fear. 'Mrs Woodrow,' I said, 'there's absolutely no reason why you can't look after another dog. You have good neighbours who can arrange walks if you can't do it yourself, and if you become incapable of looking after the dog you can give it to me and I will take personal responsibility.'

As it happened I knew of just the dog for her. As part of my job I had to visit Battersea Dogs' Home every week where a lovely little Jack Russell type dog had been abandoned in late pregnancy. Muffin, as she had been christened by the staff, had five pups a few days later. She was a good mum and all the pups were homed without difficulty, but no one seemed interested in Muffin. After four months she was looking miserable. The only person to whom she would respond was Bridget, one of the kennelmaids. When Bridget was around Muffin would wag her tail and stand at the front of her cage waiting to be petted. The rest of the time she languished at the back, showing little interest in the potential new owners who poured through the home each day. Hardly the best way to sell yourself! Yet she was a gentle, loving dog, and ideal, I thought, for Mrs Woodrow. So I fixed up a meeting.

Muffin sat in a despondent heap at the back of the cage, and Mrs Woodrow was at first uncertain until Bridget told her of how the dog had been abandoned, had had pups and was just pining for a nice home. There were forms to fill in and the Home had to be satisfied that somebody would exercise Muffin twice daily and be at home with her. Finally Muffin trotted out on a brand new lead tasting freedom and a new life.

A week later I checked her in the surgery to see how she was settling in. It was obvious from the way she skipped into the surgery and the lovely smile on Mrs Woodrow's face that things were going well. The only sad person was Bridget, who had burst into tears when Muffin left and kept her identity tag as a memento.

From time to time, I would see Muffin and her owner in the surgery – mostly for minor ailments or booster vaccinations – and nearly four years flew by. Then, one Monday morning, I had a phone call to tell me the sad news that Mrs Woodrow had died the previous week, and that she had asked for Muffin to be brought to me for rehoming. Muffin might have ended up as a friend for my own dog, Barney, except that by chance my next-door neighbour Peggy had recently lost her dog. I thought she must be feeling lonely without one.

By coincidence she had been meaning to ask me about finding another dog and Muffin fitted in perfectly. Right from the start I knew they would be happy. I felt happy, too, as I had promised Mrs Woodrow that I would make sure that Muffin was all right if anything happened to her. Living next door made it easy. By this time Muffin was about five and very well trained. She and Peggy became inseparable – and, strangely enough, while living next door to me Muffin didn't suffer a day's illness. Even so, she would always look vaguely worried whenever she saw me and nip back in if she was in the garden and would always need some coaxing to come and say hello when I visited. Later I moved to north London, but stayed in regular contact and kept the vaccines up to date.

Ten years passed with Muffin in perfect health until, at the age of fifteen, she developed arthritis. For six months this responded to anti-inflammatory pills and she was able to get round the block, albeit slowly. But, as is so often the case with old animals, once things start to go wrong other things follow and decline can be rapid. Within a short time

171

it was obvious that Muffin was wearing out, and towards the end of the month I travelled to south London to bring her back to the hospital for tests. These showed that her kidneys and liver were failing, in addition to the arthritis which was no longer responding to treatment. Her quality of life was not good and I couldn't offer more than perhaps a little improvement short term. Both Peggy and I were choked up. Muffin had come to the end of a happy fourteen years with two wonderful, caring owners, after a very uncaring start to life. I suppose there was a lot to celebrate, really, but putting her to sleep upset me even though I knew I was ultimately fulfilling a promise I had made eleven years before.

As October came towards its end the bangs started – we were nearing the Guy Fawkes season. No longer one or even a few nights, it is now degenerating into nearly a month of late-night noisy fireworks, which cause no end of misery for some pets and their owners. There, at the beginning of a busy afternoon session, were Daisy and Prince Boy. This time she was not exaggerating – anyone could see that the poor dog was a lot more apprehensive than usual. One of the other dogs barked at him and he jumped like a nervous racehorse. He sat shivering mournfully as though he had a fever. A quick check established that nothing was wrong: it was an acute case of 'nerves' brought on by the noise of the last few days. Prince Boy had taken to trembling at the bottom of Daisy's bed and wasn't getting enough sleep. Apparently he had been upset last year but this was worse and had probably been brought on by a neighbouring family with unruly teenagers who were in the habit of letting off bangers all the time. Daisy's complaints had been ignored so she had come to the hospital hoping that Prince Boy could have a sedative injection. She was rather hoping he could have one every day.

'I think the best idea is to have a small number of pills and give him half to one of them when the noise starts. There will be some days when it rains and you probably won't need them,' I suggested. The dog would need regular sedation for perhaps three weeks, which was more than I would have liked, but looking at his anxious face I knew that it would have to be. Daisy set off for home with a week's supply, and we would see how effective they were before I prescribed any more. She was the first of many in a similar plight.

Towards the end of the month we had a lucky escape, thanks to Helen's good judgement. She was just going off duty when an inspector arrived with a box. Apparently it had been seen floating down a London canal. An intrepid member of the public had retrieved it, opened it and found a snake, which, terrifyingly, rattled. A *rattlesnake*! Sensibly she shut the lid right away and called the RSPCA. The inspector's plan was to get it to the Harmsworth to see if anything was wrong with it and then find a home for it, perhaps through one of the reptile associations which help us out all the time.

When the inspector arrived Helen went over to the van just to see if it was an emergency and if she needed to stay on. As they were speaking an ominous rattle came from within the box.

'No way we're having that in here!' she said, and a few phone calls later London Zoo had kindly agreed to take it off our hands. It turned out to be an eastern diamond-back rattlesnake – the tenth most venomous in the world and *the* most venomous in the United States. The consequences of it being let loose in London didn't bear thinking about and whoever had abandoned it was totally irresponsible. Talking later to Mark Martin, an inspector with a detailed knowledge of snakes, I was told that it wasn't uncommon for people to keep poisonous snakes under special licence, but even harmless snakes worry me and I can't bring myself to handle them. I was very glad Helen had been on duty and not me!

NOVEMBER

At the beginning of the month I was immensely cheered by a return visit from Joe, the exuberant Staffie. He had now been in training for six weeks and what a difference! His owner, Jeannie, had learned to become dominant and the amazing thing was how quickly Joe had accepted – even welcomed – the new arrangement. All aspects of his life were now under Jeannie's control. His walks were regular, at times that suited Jeannie, and with the help of a Halti (a special head-collar/halter that fits round the dog's nose) Joe no longer pulled when out on walks. He had learned to come, sit, lie down, stay and all the other things that well-behaved dogs can do, based on a consistent programme of firmness and reward for good behaviour and ignoring bad behaviour. I barely recognized the cheerful but obedient dog sitting on the examination table. Jeannie was happy too, and the pair had become best friends. From being a burden to everyone (I suspect even to himself) he had become a family pet.

Jeannie had had to learn to be tough at first by not allowing Joe always to get his own way. One of the first things was not to allow him on the furniture, unless he was invited. He had been occasionally confined to one room – much to his disgust, although he learned quickly to accept it – to teach him not to follow her about constantly. Whenever he tried to initiate a walk, a meal or a play, he was ignored. He had to learn that Jeannie would decide when such things happened and she would tell him to come to her and sit first. It had been hard work, though, with lots of coaching from the dog-behaviour expert.

The bangs and crashes of late October continued and reached a crescendo as 5 November approached. In the outside clinics and the hospital it was the same story: an increased number of worried owners requesting tranquillizers for Bonfire Night. This year it seemed even worse than usual and I hoped that we wouldn't see any accidents and injuries. In recent years the worst had been a dog called Cracker, who had run away from bangers thrown at him and been hit by a car, resulting in a broken jaw. In previous years I have seen injured or burned dogs and cats, and hedgehogs caught in the bonfire, quite a common place for a hedgehog to rest. The woodpile should always be checked for their presence before it is lit.

Prince Boy's medication seemed to be doing the trick and I was happy to dispense another week of pills. He walked in, a bit slower than usual, and snoozed while he was waiting to be seen, in spite of being surrounded by other dogs, cats and all manner of exotic pets. Daisy had had to cut down on his walks and there was already a hint of belly appearing.

'Watch his weight, Daisy,' I remarked, and then wished I hadn't. I had just given her something more to worry about! We weighed him, at 25.4 kilos, which was just a little more than ideal. We would put him on the scales every time he came in and adjust his diet accordingly. Although we don't do it, some vets run weight-watcher clinics for their patients, a good idea since obesity in animals can be the forerunner of many diseases, such as joint and leg problems, arthritis, diabetes, liver and heart disease.

In spite of the build-up, night duty on 5 November was

quiet. Most people, at least in our area, had heeded numerous warnings from all the animal charities to keep their pets in and well away from the fireworks. As I heard the bangs, saw the flashes and listened to the fire-engine sirens near home, I thought that the whole thing was absolute madness. Goodness knows how many children and animals, both wild and domesticated, would be injured tonight – not to mention the innumerable fires destroying property.

Another difficulty we experience at this time of year is an upsurge in the number of lost and abandoned animals coming into the hospital. I can only imagine that many stray cats and dogs have become disoriented with all the noise and failed to find their way home. More puzzling is the increase in abandoned animals: there are almost as many as during the post-Christmas period when unwanted pet presents are thrown out, and at the height of summer, when animals are dumped while their owners go on holiday.

Ward seven was full, with a mixture of very young cats, mostly unneutered males, and very old ones, the two categories of cat I would expect to be upset and confused by fireworks. The sad thing is that experience has shown that the majority of these cats would not be reclaimed. Just as in the summer, the reports nurse would be phoning round all the homing centres. If we were unsuccessful I might have to reschedule some of the non-urgent surgery cases while waiting for the cages to become free. There were only four owned cats in the ward and, of these, three were not fit to go home. They had all suffered road traffic accidents, had broken bones and needed intensive nursing. The other was Trixie, who had had an operation to remove a polyp from her throat. This is a fascinating condition, which I can't remember diagnosing in my first few years as a vet but which I have seen quite frequently in the last ten years.

177

Trixie had seen Bairbre a few days ago with noisy breathing. Her owner, Jane, a student, had at first put it down to a cold but after a couple of weeks had brought the cat in. Trixie was just over a year old and was fully vaccinated. There was no sneezing or any sign of illness except for a snuffling noise when she breathed in. At night she snored loudly. Bairbre suspected a polyp right from the start and booked Trixie in for an examination under anaesthetic. You have to be a bit careful with the anaesthetic as the cat sometimes stops breathing with the obstruction in the airway so a tube is put into the windpipe. With Trixie asleep the polyp was easy to find at the back of the pharynx. Bairbre grasped it with forceps and, with a gentle tug, brought it out completely. It is so simple, yet satisfying and fun to do. Best of all is that, within twenty-four hours, the cat is usually cured and ready to go home.

On my ward rounds I saw Trixie sitting in the top right-hand corner cage purring loudly. I had to pick her up and put her on the examination table to get her to stop purring and then listen to her breathing. It was silent and easy – a tremendous contrast to yesterday. She would probably not suffer from this problem again. The cause of these polyps is a mystery except that they often seem to originate in the middle ear and pass down the Eustachian tube, which links the ear with the back of the throat.

A disease common in London dogs is chronic bronchitis. Chalky, a ten-year-old West Highland White, was a classic case. For a start he was well overweight, tipping the scales at 15 kilos. Obesity is known to make chronic bronchitis worse: the heart has difficulty in pumping blood round a fat body and congested lungs. Chalky lived in a built-up area with the nearest park more than a mile away. Little dogs near to the ground are prone to suffer from the pollution of car exhaust and I was quite sure that this was a major factor. As well as this, Bob and Ethel, his owners, and their grown up son Jim who was still at home, were all smokers which could only make matters worse.

Over the last two years Chalky had been in with a cough that cleared up on treatment then relapsed some months later. The relapses had become more frequent and he had been booked in for a chest X-ray. I was worried about giving him an anaesthetic as he was so overweight and had a bad chest, so opted for deep sedation. This worked well and he almost fell asleep while I pressed the button to take the picture. These days, we are blessed with automatic developers that can process X-ray film in less than five minutes so I was able to see what was going on inside his chest right away.

There was little doubt about it. Chalky's lungs had been substantially damaged by years of pollution. Going over the X-ray later that day with the family, I had to draw the fine line between getting the message across and preaching. That's quite hard for me, a rabid anti-smoker! I pointed out the thickening of the main airways and the general congestion in the lung tissue and warned them that the damage was probably permanent. 'His best chance lies with a three-pronged attack. First, he needs to lose weight, second, we have to control the inflammation, and last, try to ensure that he doesn't have any infection,' I told them, adding that he would need antibiotics, low-dose steroids and a crash diet. Then I got on to the difficult bit. 'But, of course, if we can't keep him away from smoke then we're really wasting our time.'

This was taken on board quickly. Within a minute the whole family had decided to give up smoking. Years of warnings and admonishments from the family GP had

179

fallen on deaf ears, but since the dog was suffering – well, that was different. Although I have never smoked myself I know how difficult it is to stop since I see some of the nurses going through it periodically. Just two have genuinely succeeded in the last year.

Chalky was discharged on antibiotics, less than half rations, some steroids and a drug called aminophylline, which helps to dilate the airways. If we were going to see an improvement it should be within a month. With Christmas coming up I thought that the stop-smoking campaign might come under strain, but I found myself looking forward to seeing the dog and his family again for an update on how they were all coping and especially whether Chalky was improving.

We always see an increase in coughing animals at this time of year as viruses abound in winter, and the damp, cold November days seem to make things worse. For this reason, chronic bronchitis is often bad in the winter. In many cases, it only improves with the dry, warmer days of early summer.

It's not just dogs, cats and humans who suffer from a smoky atmosphere. When Helen looked at Coco, a cockatiel with an obvious wheeze, his chest puffed up and heaving respiration, it was obvious to her that he had a chest infection. For most vets it would have been tempting just to put him on antibiotics and hope for the best. Helen, though, seems able to home in on the less obvious aspects of a case, especially when it comes to exotics. She discovered two things. Coco's diet was wrong for him: he was fed too many sunflower seeds, which are high in fat and low in vitamin A, and he was living in a very smoky atmosphere, just like Chalky, so needed similar treatment plus a change in diet.

Another case that Helen saw on the same afternoon delighted me in its simplicity, and I wondered whether I would have picked up so quickly on the diagnosis. Stumpy, a three-legged hamster, was presented with a swelling on the right side of his face. He had had a chequered history, having to have his leg amputated when he broke it badly aged six months. Now, nearing two, he was entering old age for a hamster. I would have immediately thought an abscess was the cause of the swelling, but Helen had noticed that the swelling was on the same side as the stump. She put gentle pressure on the swelling and out came a load of impacted food. The other cheek pouch was empty. The answer was simple: Stumpy had not been able to massage the pouch because he didn't have a leg on that side! Apparently hamsters tend to use their hind legs to squeeze out food stuck in their pouches. Now his owners would have to do this for him.

Later that day I searched through my books on hamsters to see what was said on pouch impaction but didn't find much. What I did read, however, was that the word hamster comes from the German 'to hoard' and that hamster means 'hoarder'. And that the most common cause of pouch impaction is the hamster being given sticky sweets by a child – which I had never come across.

In the afternoon clinic I saw another equally simple, common condition. Petra, an English bull terrier, had been mated with a dog of the same breed a few months before and her owners had been eagerly awaiting the arrival of some pups. The children were keen to see the magic of their birth and rearing. There hadn't been any signs to suggest that anything might be wrong. Petra had started to eat more than usual, had put on weight, her mammary glands had filled out and in the last few days had begun to produce milk.

The whole family trooped into the consulting room,

Mum, Dad and the children, Michael and Katie. According to Katie, who had been counting off the days, Petra had been due to give birth yesterday but instead of getting on with the job she had become morose and had gone round the house picking up various objects and transferring them to her bed. These were now put on display. A pair of swimming goggles, a rubber duck, a fluffy toy, Po – one of the Teletubbies – and a spectacle case. She had arranged these objects in her bed, nuzzling them and moving them about. Meanwhile, she was off her food.

I suspected that Petra was suffering from false pregnancy in an extreme form. She had even turned possessive about her 'pups' and growled at me when I tried to move them out of the way to examine her tummy. A gentle prod and it was pretty obvious that although there was lots of milk – enough for six pups – there were no pups. False pregnancy is the result of a hormonal imbalance and affected bitches tend to have the problem after each season. In later life, they are also much more at risk from developing pyometra, an infected womb. Our general recommendation is to clear up the milk with drugs, then operate to remove the womb and ovaries.

Petra's family were gloomy as I told them this – they had been so looking forward to the 'event', which looked now as though it would never happen. 'You can always try again,' I said. 'But she may be that little bit more difficult to get into pup, as you have already found out.'

Breeding dogs is really best done by the specialists who do everything they can to ensure the best for their breed. Petra was on the small side, and might have had difficulty in giving birth anyway. I prescribed some pills to reduce the milk and suggested that her 'pups' be removed gradually over the next week. The presence of the toys would probably stimulate more milk but to take them all away suddenly struck me as unkind. The family would think about having her spayed.

The owner of Toffee, a four-year-old mongrel bitch, which I saw in the same session, was going to get similar advice but for a different reason. She was in season now and had managed to scale a six-foot fence in the garden and had been last seen disappearing over the hill with three male dogs. She was missing for eight hours and came in with her tail between her legs, in a sorry state of exhaustion. She had eaten her evening meal then collapsed into her bed and slept it off. This was not the first time she had escaped: in two previous seasons she had once jumped out of the car, when it stopped at traffic lights, and once over the garden fence. As a result, she had had two litters of pups. In spite of this, her owner, Lisa, a single parent, had still not got round to having her spayed. This time she was booked in to have the operation, but for the present it would be necessary to prevent the pregnancy. This is accomplished by an injection of female hormones, which needs to be given within two or three days of the mating. A still tired-looking Toffee didn't even notice the injection and happily hopped off the table when told to. That still left the problem of getting her past the waiting room full of male dogs, who had suddenly become restless. We went out of the back door into the car-park. While I watched, Lisa bundled Toffee into the car, then came back to me.

'This injection can only really be given once,' I said to her, 'so you'll have to be extra careful with Toffee!' Like many bits of advice vets hand out, this would be easier said than done and, even as I spoke, Toffee was eyeing up a largish dog trotting into the hospital with his master and not on a lead. If she got out now it would be disastrous. Lisa was about to get into the car when I pointed to the loose dog. 'Wait!' I said. Just in time Lisa shut the door. Then, after a minute, she eased herself in and drove away, with Toffee leaping about on the back seat and looking out through the rear window. Lisa would have her hands full for the next couple of weeks, and unfortunately the operation would have to wait for a month or so. Although spaying is routine and straightforward, it is not recommended to be done while the dog is in season as all the blood vessels are swollen and there is a much increased risk of bleeding.

My day was turning into an almost 100 per cent obstetrics session, and finished with an infected womb that would need removing the next day. The old Labrador was put on a drip and given antibiotics overnight in preparation for the operation.

The next morning I was in the skin clinic with a much happier Bill and Teddy. The antibiotics had seen off the secondary infection, and maybe it was that, or the build-up of the effect of the evening-primrose oil and/or the vaccine, but there was a definite and quite dramatic improvement. I turned Teddy over and looked at the hairless part of his tummy: no sign of the angry red spots, just normal, healthy pink skin. I checked out his previously itchy feet, face and armpits. They were a lot less inflamed. For the last week Teddy had not been itching at all and was a different dog, more relaxed and enjoying life. His vaccines were now just monthly and I kept up the antibiotic for another month along with the evening-primrose oil. The next check would be just before Christmas – where had the year gone?

A loud bang at one in the morning reminded me that Guy Fawkes 'night' was still going on, days after the event. It was such a loud explosion that it woke my elder daughter, no mean feat, and I had to go into her bedroom to calm her down. As is often the case, once I had woken I found it difficult to get back to sleep and was like a bear with a sore head the next day.

My mood wasn't improved by the sight of eighteen stray cats in ward seven and the news from the reports nurse that she had been able to place only six in the homing centres. On the operating list were ten cats, which would need admitting, and Sam, the wards supervisor, was scurrying round looking for free cages to put them in. It had been like this for the last three weeks but I was determined not to let it get me down. I had to admit, though, that the constant pressure was wearing and this was a problem that could be easily solved if fireworks were restricted to organized displays. And I *wish* people would get their cats microchipped!

It's amazing how common baldness is in pet animals. We see bald dogs, cats, guinea-pigs, gerbils, rats, mice and hamsters. For the most part it doesn't bother the affected animal but the owners worry terribly. Maybe this is an extension of the worry they would feel if they were to lose their own hair. Hammy was a balding hamster brought in by his ten-year-old owner with his mum for moral support.

'His hair's gone all wispy,' said Joe, 'and you can see the wrinkled skin underneath.'

Baldness is common in hamsters and is usually caused by *Demodex*, the same mite that caused Heidi's problem. With hamsters, though, there are two different species of mite, *Demodex aurati* and *Demodex criceti*. One is long and thin, the other is short and stumpy. This is the sort of thing that delights parasitologists, who can spend hours peering at them down their microscopes. Rolf Harris had seen his first hamster *Demodex* the day before with Bairbre in a virtually identical case to the one I was examining now. I can well remember his first view of a mite. It was *Sarcoptes scabiei*, from a dog with scabies, and he immediately drew a cartoon of the dog and Sir Coptes Mite!

Just as in Heidi's case I would have to do skin scrapings to try to capture one of Hammy's mites. I found his biggest bald patch and scraped away. A few minutes later, I was rewarded with a view under the microscope of the slender, cigar-shaped *Demodex aurati*. If only all cases were so straightforward! The drawback was that the disease in hamsters is usually associated with old age, which makes the long-term outlook poor. As the hamster becomes old its immune system fails and it can no longer keep the *Demodex* mite at bay. The result is a big increase in their numbers, which damages the hairs – just as it does in the dog. But it's always worth trying treatment and hoping for an extra six months of life. I explained all this to Joe, who had read about it anyway in his hamster book. He was determined that Hammy, who was two and a half, would live until he was at least three, which is about the hamster's natural life-span. He would have to bath Hammy in the same shampoo used to treat Heidi, but in a more dilute form.

Mum said hardly a word throughout but she was obviously proud of her caring son, who listened carefully to everything I said and would, no doubt, follow all instructions to the letter.

By far the commonest mite is the ear mite, and I had it in mind to find a cat with them and catch some. Usually we don't bother to put them under the microscope because they are quite easy to see with the naked eye and that's all that is necessary to make a diagnosis. However, they are quite fascinating to look at under a microscope, with long legs and intricate suckers at the end of each. The mite is called *Otodectes cynotis* and is common in kittens. With the naked eye they look like tiny white dots about the size of a pinhead. They move around at great speed and cause tremendous irritation, with much head-shaking and scratching.

I didn't have long to wait before a suitable case came through the door: a young female tortoiseshell with the usual symptoms. Just a simple swab of the ear was all that was needed to catch some mites. For Rolf and much of the film crew, this was the first time they had seen the bizarre-looking creature and opinion was roughly divided between repulsion and fascination.

A cat I saw the next day would have been much more interesting in television terms, but this was a Friday afternoon when little filming is done as everyone winds down for the weekend. Fifi came in looking intensely miserable. Her face was itchy and her eyes were swollen. She had started to rub her face and eyes just a few days before and her owner, a retired caretaker, had decided to come in because he didn't want to leave things as they were over the weekend. Just as well he did, because once cats start attacking themselves in this way it only takes them a few days to make a right mess of themselves.

There are only a few diagnoses that fitted Fifi's symptoms. Allergy, like hay-fever, is one, food allergy another and allergy to ear mites is the third. With Fifi I thought immediately of allergy to ear mites, because she had had an ear problem for a few weeks and now it had suddenly got much worse. Unlike my tortoiseshell of the day before, finding a mite in the allergy situation is difficult: many have been scratched or rubbed off due to the intense irritation. But, as luck would have it, I found a solitary *Otodectes* on Fifi's rump. This is a good place to look for them: when the cat goes to sleep the tail is near the ears and the mites meander on to it. Treatment is simple: a shot of steroid to reduce the irritation, and a blitzkrieg on the mites with ear drops

187

and all-over shampooing. Fortunately Fifi was one of those easy-going laid-back cats that enjoyed baths. She would probably be cured quickly and I didn't expect to see her again. It made a nice end to the week.

The following Monday it seemed that the firework pressure was off. The bangs had receded and most of the stray cats had somehow been found homing centres. Filming had been going on since September but, for the most part, we could forget it was happening because the crews would be concentrated in one consulting room or the operating theatre. The rest of the hospital just got on with its routine work.

Everyone, including Rolf, was pleased to see Heidi in for her first check-up. Phil was coping splendidly with the hard work – Heidi was one lucky dog. She was doing well and the nasty sores were healing quite nicely. She wasn't itchy and was finding her natural doggy joy of living again. She bounded in with much wagging, trying to lick everyone. Although she was still nearly bald there was more than a hint of fine hair coming through in most places. This cheered me no end because the risk is great in neglected cases of the hair follicles being destroyed. If that had happened, Heidi would have remained bald. She and Phil went out armed with another month's worth of treatment. The next time I saw them would be just before Christmas. As usual I hadn't bought any presents yet, and a twinge of panic shot through me! No time to think of that for the moment, though, not with all these animals pouring through the door.

One cat which had excited attention was a white Persian called Snowdrop which had gone missing for six weeks. There is nothing worse for a cat owner than their pet's disappearance. In some ways it's worse than the cat dying because at least that way they know what has happened. It's the not knowing that causes the anguish. I've had this happen with a couple of cats but never for more than a few days and six weeks is a very long time: most owners would have given up the search. John and Lucy never lost hope. They had done all the usual things, such as ringing the RSPCA, the local vets, other cat charities, had put up notices in the area and gone round all the neighbours asking them to check their garages. For six weeks, though, they had no luck – and then Snowdrop turned up on her owners' doorstep, a very different Snowdrop. The once beautifully silky coat was dirty, matted and flea-ridden, and she was much thinner than before, although that would not be obvious until she was examined at the hospital.

Matting of the fur is particularly associated with long-haired cats. They need a lot of grooming, preferably at least half an hour per day. Most of the problems I see are in temperamental cats like Snowdrop. What cats get up to during the day is a mystery – they probably don't stray too far but, being curious, there is plenty of opportunity for them to get into mischief, with fights, accidents and getting shut in sheds. No one could tell what had happened to Snowdrop but her disappearance had coincided with the onset of the firework season so perhaps she had been frightened and disoriented.

The solution was to give her an anaesthetic and clip off all the mats. She would end up with something like a crew-cut and John and Lucy were warned that she would look a complete mess afterwards. We have learned to warn people of the results of de-matting because otherwise they think we can tease out the mats and restore the beauty of the cat like magic. Afterwards only Snowdrop's face had normal hair on it. She was under the anaesthetic for three-quarters of an hour before all the mats were off. Then she had to be wrapped up in a blanket to conserve her heat. It would be four or five months before she had a fully glossy coat once more. In spite of her appearance, though, John and Lucy were delighted to have her back and to know that all she needed now was lots of TLC.

We see many quite normal, healthy animals in the surgery, often because without experience of a particular breed it is hard to know what *is* normal. For example, I remember seeing my first ever Chinese crested dog and thinking it had some serious hormonal deficiency. It was only while chatting to the owner that she let slip, 'Of course, these dogs are naturally bald – but I don't have to tell *you* that.'

'Of course,' I lied, and made a mental note to read up about the breed.

Devon or Cornish Rex cats can be a bit of a challenge to anyone not familiar with them. They are charming creatures, with sparse, crinkly hair. And some animals have glands, which are quite normal but when first noticed may precipitate a trip to the vet.

Jamie the hamster had been rushed in right at the end of the afternoon clinic. Strictly speaking his owner, Susie, a student, was too late for this session but Terry the receptionist asked if I would fit the hamster in as Susie was so worried. Jamie was eighteen months old – in his prime – and Susie had noticed dark patches on each of his flanks. They were a bit moist and covered in coarser hair than the rest of the flank. Susie was convinced that they were growths: someone who apparently knew about hamsters had told her that they were probably melanomas. Susie knew that melanomas can be malignant and spread all over the body, so she plucked up courage and came in to the hospital expecting the worst.

190

It's true that hamsters can suffer from malignant tumours, such as melanoma, along with many other animals. But Jamie's problem wasn't a problem at all. On either side of a hamster there is an area of specialized glandular tissue called the hip or scent gland. They seem to have a function in marking territory and also in mating because they are prominent in males during the mating season. All that Jamie was doing was proclaiming to the hamster world that he was male and available!

Learning about all the normal things to do with animals is enormous fun but daunting, and keeping up-to-date with the diseases of dogs and cats is a huge task, let alone learning all about the normal biology of other animal species. Small domesticated rodents are a growth area in veterinary medicine at the moment, and I am looking forward to going on courses over the next few years to learn more about them. I felt sorry for Susie, who had rushed in in great anxiety only to be told that her pet was entirely normal. She was relieved but felt a bit foolish. Still, as I pointed out to her, it's better to ask for advice sooner rather than later.

At the end of the month came the excellent news that the balcony-dogs cruelty case had come to court. The owner had been found guilty, had been made to pay a substantial fine and, most importantly, had been banned from keeping dogs. Best of all, the dogs had all been found excellent homes.

DECEMBER

Bowser was in terrible pain. He had gone off his food, unusual for a Boxer, and he couldn't open his right eye. He couldn't bear anyone to go near it either. This had come on overnight, and he was sitting in the waiting room when I arrived at eight-fifteen on the first morning of the month. He was whining and pawing at his eye and it was obvious that no one would be able to make a proper examination without knocking him out. He would be admitted and dealt with as a priority.

Meanwhile Jenny, the admissions nurse, was trying to get some more information from his worried owners about how the eye might have been damaged. The only thing they could think was that Hatfield, a feisty tortoiseshell kitten, and a new addition to the family, might have scratched the dog. But Richard and Sheila couldn't believe that she would have caused such damage – Bowser had accepted her right from the start and she was often to be found sleeping in his basket with him. But at only a year he wasn't much older than the cat and the two of them spent hours cavorting about. An accidental scratch seemed possible.

It turned out to be me who got to look at him. The ward rounds were short for a change and by the time I'd finished Bowser had been given a sedative. However, it was slow to take effect and he was still jumping about. Nevertheless, within ten seconds of injecting the anaesthetic thiopentone into his vein he was slumbering out flat on the table. Using special forceps to open his eyelids wide it was immediately apparent that he had sustained a nasty laceration to the cornea. No doubt about it, it was a cat scratch and a pretty bad one. No wonder his eye was all screwed up. There was a real danger that he could lose the sight in it. If the cornea ruptured, the iris would prolapse through and glaucoma (an increase in the pressure within the eye) might result.

The laceration had not quite gone through the entire cornea, which was a hopeful sign. The first thing to do was to dilate the eye. This would minimize the risk of the iris prolapsing through if the cornea ruptured. But how to prevent the rupture? Fortunately there exists a fairly common procedure which we use in situations like this. Dogs and cats have a third eyelid which can just be seen in the corner of their eyes. With gentle pulling, under anaesthesia of course, this can be made to cover the entire eye then stitched into place, either through the upper lid or into the white part of the eye, where it acts as a corneal bandage. Usually this technique works well – but only time would tell.

As in all these urgent cases the owners had to play the waiting game. For Richard and Sheila it was difficult because they had a three-year-old son who was very attached to the dog and would have to be kept well away for the next ten days or so. If the eye couldn't be saved it would put a dampener on Christmas, which was now only a few weeks off. As he came round from his relatively short anaesthetic the usually irrepressible Bowser looked a sorry sight. To add insult to injury, he would need to wear an Elizabethan collar for the next ten days, to prevent him scratching his eye while it was healing, but at least with the benefit of modern pain-killers he should soon be feeling more comfortable.

December is always a special month in the Animal

Hospital's year. It always seems to go so quickly – although in our business all the months fly by. We had had cameras around for over three months in the current series of the television programme. Their presence also seemed to make the time go even faster. I have not been able to work out why – perhaps it's the frenetic energy which programme production always generates. It seemed to have been less stressful this time round and we had all developed ways of letting it interfere as little as possible. My strategy had been to keep out of the camera's eye except when wanted. Where the filming goes on is always a mass of cables and crew, but the next room would usually be functioning as usual and could as easily be hundreds of miles away.

The Christmas tree went up and the cards started to flood in but no one seemed to notice that the workload showed no sign of easing as the festive season approached.

One welcome visitor in for a check-up was Heidi. Right from the moment she burst into the consulting room, almost tripping over the cameras, we could see that she had improved (literally) in leaps and bounds. In December Heidi was full of the joys of spring. She had also made friends with Phil's other dog, Boris, although this had its downside, as Phil told me. Heidi, of course, had probably never known what it was to have a proper, caring home and had learned to be street-wise. She couldn't be trusted to leave food alone. No surprise, I suppose: whether you're a dog or a human, if you don't know where your next meal is coming from you tend to eat when food is available. In short, Heidi was a food thief, and she had turned the talents of her new friend to her advantage. As Phil put it, 'Boris opens the fridge and Heidi empties it!'

Apart from this, everything was going so well. Heidi's hair was growing through thick and fast and there was no

195

irritation or redness in her skin. I knew that it would take at least another three months for the hair to come back completely, and that we would have to carry on with the treatment, but I was looking forward to seeing a beautiful glossy coat and comparing the photos with the original desperate condition in which she had been found – my turn to be patient.

Much of veterinary practice is routine and the common ailments crop up time and time again, but whenever a bizarre or rare condition appears it makes my day. Pemphigus is a condition in which the body attacks its own tissue with antibodies. Such conditions are called autoimmune diseases. Pemphigus is also seen in people in the form of skin blisters – which is where the name comes from: it is from the Greek, meaning blister. In dogs and cats, though, it is much more inclined to produce crusts on various parts of the skin. In animals the first case was described in 1975 in a dog, by an American vet called Tony Stannard. Since then many cases have been seen in dogs, cats and other species, and we expect to treat maybe two or three cases a year in the hospital. I had been qualified seven years before pemphigus was described, which makes it a fair bet that I had seen it and not known what I was looking at, although searching through my memory banks I couldn't recall such a case in my early days.

Now it was Helen's turn to see a cat with this strange condition. Poppy was a four-year-old moggy, which had developed the signs of one type of the disease called *Pemphigus foliaceus*. Poppy's ears were very crusty in particular, and would become increasingly so, then ulcerated and painful. It's sometimes possible to find scabs elsewhere on the body, round the nose and on the footpads, for example. Poppy had the lot. The great thing with this disease in cats is that it usually responds well to treatment but first Helen needed confirmation of the diagnosis by sending a small slice of skin to the laboratory for the histopathologist to examine. This is absolutely necessary, because the treatment would involve very high doses of steroids. Poppy's owners were concerned but Helen was hopeful that all would end well and quicker than they thought – perhaps even by Christmas. The poor cat's ears were so crusty and sore that it didn't seem possible. The next day, after her biopsy had been done, Poppy was on her way home. Helen had requested a fax report, so with a bit of luck we would have to wait only a few days before we got confirmation and then the treatment could begin.

Towards the middle of the month Bowser was back, looking a lot less miserable. Another quick anaesthetic, stitches out and, thank goodness, the cornea was healing well. He might be left with a small scar on the cornea but his sight in the eye was going to be fine. He had even learned to be a bit more cautious with the kitten. Thinking about it, over the years I couldn't remember seeing a dog that had suffered the same fate twice. There was much joy in the Bowser household as they came to pick him up and found out that not only was the eye saved but that he wouldn't have to wear the collar anymore. Just another week or two of ointment in Bowser's eye to make sure no infection could linger, and in the final entry on his card I put BIW – back if worried. I didn't expect to see him again, though – barring accidents, and the natural tendency for exuberant Boxers to have them!

Accidents are an unfortunate feature of every vet's life, particularly in busy hospitals, and I suppose there is hardly a worse time for a much-loved pet to suffer a life-threatening mishap than in December. But, unfortunately, this is one of those months when they seem to happen often – perhaps it's down to the long dark evenings. Cats outnumber dogs by far when it comes to accidents. Of their injuries, pelvic fractures are the most common and we average four or five patients hospitalized every week for this. Other fractures occur too, but once we get accident cases into the hospital they have a reasonable chance of survival.

Tom, a young male cat, was being looked at by Bairbre in the prep room. He had life-threatening injuries. Shocked and with breathing difficulties, he needed a chest X-ray fairly fast. The three commonest chest injuries we see after accidents are haemorrhage into the chest, air entering the chest from a wound, which causes the lungs to collapse, and rupture of the diaphragm. Any of these may cause the death of the animal and the third, rupture of the diaphragm, requires major surgery, which is not always successful.

With fluids dripping into his veins to counteract the shock and pain-killers taking effect, Tom was gently restrained with padded weights while an X-ray was taken of his chest. Two minutes later, Bairbre had her diagnosis: Tom's diaphragm was ruptured. The diaphragm is the muscle that separates the chest from the abdomen and ruptures following a severe blow to the abdomen, usually from a car. Quite often, part of the liver, or sometimes all of it, passes through into the chest. When that happens some of the intestines follow too. This had happened to Tom because on the X-ray Bairbre could see loops of intestine near his heart. This was a more severe case than usual and Tom's life hung in the balance. Because of his breathing difficulty he would need life-saving surgery as soon as he was fit to stand the anaesthetic: it was scheduled for the following morning.

First thing the next day, Bairbre and a team of experienced nurses set about the task of trying to sort out the young cat's problems. Having spent a little time in an oxygen tent, Tom was given an injection into his vein to make him unconscious. Then a tube was inserted into his lungs and connected to the anaesthetic machine through which gas would be passed to keep him asleep during the operation. All the fur had been clipped away and the initial incision was made into his abdomen. This is one of the critical parts of the operation because as soon as the abdomen is opened the cat can no longer breathe on his own and a machine has to do it for him. At this point he may die. But the team got past it and the rupture in the diaphragm was localized. With gentle tugging, the liver and loops of intestine were brought back to their right places and the laborious, meticulous repair of the diaphragm could begin.

All went well to start with, and then Tom's pulse got weaker. Without further warning, his heart stopped. Frantic efforts were made to revive him with an injection of heart stimulants and direct massage. Just when all seemed lost, it started again. Bairbre redoubled her efforts and soon completed the repair. Another critical phase in the operation came now: would Tom start to breathe on his own? A few minutes later, the team had their answer when Tom made his first faltering but determined efforts to get air into his lungs. Even now he was not yet out of the woods: there was a danger of fluid build-up and he needed a chest drain to be inserted. This took another ten minutes and then bloody fluid was sucked out of his chest. This made his breathing easier and, for the first time since his accident, his tongue looked a healthy pink.

Now he would have twenty-four hours of intensive treatment, with frequent checks of his breathing and drain plus pain-killers and a drip. In the last ninety minutes he had

199

lost more than half of his nine lives – but having got him this far the outlook was much better. There was an air of quiet jubilation among the team. The whole procedure had been filmed too, and a few days later ten million people would have the opportunity to watch the tremendous efforts that had been made to ensure that one very lucky cat lived.

Once cats enter the recovery phase, progress is rapid. A day later Tom was sitting up in his cage with a calm look on his face as if to say, 'What's all the fuss about?' He would make it for sure now – in fact in a few weeks' time, no doubt, he would be enjoying his turkey like millions of other cats. His owners, an elderly couple, didn't find out about the drama until it was all over. They were horrified to hear what had happened to him but happy to have him home and recovering for Christmas.

In the run-up to Christmas the pace inevitably slackens. People are shopping for presents or, if they are like me, worrying about what to get. This is one time of the year when we do have an opportunity to take stock and plan ahead. Most of the surgery we perform is on emergency cases because most of the non-urgent operations will be planned for January.

However, Harry, a tough little Yorkie, had been brought forward on the list because his leg problem had got worse. Harry had something quite common, a dislocating knee cap. It's so easily identified when you've seen it for the first time: the dog walks along normally for half a dozen paces then hops on three legs for another half-dozen before getting back to normal again. The diagnosis is easy: push out the knee cap then immediately replace it! This makes the owners go green, although most dogs just sit there and let you do it. Harry was now hopping more than walking normally.

One morning, between cases, I popped into the small theatre to see Gabriel and watched, fascinated, while he deftly sorted out Harry's sliding knee cap. He had to make the groove in which Harry's knee cap lay a little deeper so that it couldn't slip out. If this isn't done, arthritis sets in eventually and the dog is in constant pain. Using a fine oscillating bone saw, Gabriel cut a triangular groove in the cartilage where the knee cap lies and removed it, setting it to one side. Then, using the saw again, he deepened the groove, put the bit of cartilage back then replaced the knee cap. Almost an instant cure, although Harry would have to wait until the new year before playing football, his favourite pastime, with the two young boys in his family. I must try that next time, I thought. But it would have to wait until after Christmas – I had to get down to the serious business of buying presents.

Talking of presents, Teddy's owner, Bill, came in with some chocolates for the nurses and much appreciated they were too. Meanwhile, Teddy looked completely normal and was in remission from his severe allergies. We could stop the antibiotics and see how he coped without them. Life would be much simpler with just a couple of evening-primrose oil capsules each evening and a monthly vaccine. But, as I warned Bill, 'It might not last. In fact, to tell you the truth, it probably won't. This is one disease which keeps waxing and waning.' But I hoped to keep on top of it, for Teddy's sake. The difference in him was lovely to see. The best thing was that we knew exactly what was wrong with him and that is always half the battle. I do hate it when we never get to the bottom of things.

Somehow I wasn't surprised that Prince Boy was in again with Daisy – she was convinced this time he had a cold. He was off his food and coughing and gagging. As if to prove it he produced a theatrical little splutter right on cue.

'See?' said Daisy. 'He's got a cold!' She had never accepted that there was nothing wrong with Prince Boy on the many occasions we had told her this. Now she had been proven right! I took his temperature, which was normal, and he didn't seem unwell except for the little cough and somewhat exaggerated swallowing. I tried to get a decent look at his tonsils but he wasn't having any of it. As a last resort before I had to admit him for a full anaesthetic I gave him a sedative jab and sent him out into the waiting room – I'd have another go in ten minutes.

As he went off with Daisy I caught sight of Mrs Fortuna walking up the rows dispensing advice and sympathy in equal quantities. 'Where's Mr Harry?' I said, with a questioning frown.

'He's at home,' she replied. 'I'm just here to give Daisy moral support.' I suppose I shouldn't have been surprised that they were friends but, anyway, I was too busy to discuss it with her now. We were running behind, and Prince Boy might need an anaesthetic. I got on with the usual run-of-the-mill cases in outpatients, tummy upsets, anal-sac blockages, ear problems and so on before getting Daisy into the clinic again.

The sedative had done the trick. We lifted Prince Boy on to the table where he promptly settled down with both eyes shut. Every now and then he would open them to check if I was still there and then, realizing that I was, he would shut them again with a sigh. I waited a few minutes until I was sure he was relaxed, then gingerly opened his jaws. There, stuck at the back, was a piece of rib bone. It neatly traversed the whole of the roof of his mouth and must have been very irritating, although I couldn't see any inflammation. I picked up some forceps, opened the dog's mouth again, grabbed the bone and pulled it out. Prince Boy gave another theatrical sigh and rested his head on my arm.

'So it wasn't a cold, then?' Daisy asked. The answer, of course, was no, and she asked to take the rib bone home to show the neighbours. Prince Boy would need no further treatment. This was the first time I could remember when he had something potentially seriously wrong with him. I was very glad that I hadn't just sent him home on treatment and missed the bone altogether. Prince Boy was made of strong stuff and managed to stagger out in a slightly inebriated state.

In the waiting room I heard Mrs Fortuna advising someone on the virtues of herbal flea collars. I opened my mouth to tell her that the vets or the nurses would give out the advice around here and could she please come in only when her own animals were ill, when she caught sight of me.

'Mr Grant,' she exclaimed, 'I've got something for you.' And with that she produced a tin of biscuits and a Christmas card. Ah, well! I thanked her and wished her and Daisy a happy Christmas and New Year. They departed, with Prince Boy swaying between them.

The last few days before Christmas are among the happiest in the year, with visits from other RSPCA establishments and trips to the other clinics for their parties. The Christmas tree in the lounge looked lovely and we were now in the festive spirit. In the run-up to the holiday I was trying to get the owned animals out so that the emergency crew on Christmas Day and Boxing Day would have only a small number of strays to look after. No routine operations are booked in and I try very hard each ward rounds to get the patients home.

One of the most unusual cases we have ever had around

Christmas was seen by Bairbre. A kitten had climbed to the top of the tree and fallen off. The unlucky little thing had cracked its shin bone – a greenstick fracture. These are always seen in very young animals with thin, developing bones. Sometimes we need to put on a splint, but more often than not, if the animal is kept confined and rested, the bone will heal by itself quite quickly, in a couple of weeks.

Christmas was now upon us, and for the first time in ten years I wasn't going to be on duty on the day. As director of the hospital, I had always found it easiest to volunteer to do it myself so that the others could go home. Secretly I enjoyed my Christmas duties – it's the one day of the year when everyone is good-humoured and genuinely apologetic for interrupting your day. Over the previous nine years the day had been mostly quiet – with some notable exceptions. One year I had a gastric torsion in a standard poodle (the stomach twisted on itself and bloated), which survived an emergency operation at midnight on Christmas Eve, followed by a Caesarean on a young cat ending up with five bonny kittens. I ended up with about four hours' sleep. This year my wife put her foot down: I was wanted at home all day. In any case, Gabriel had volunteered to be on duty – in fact, he was positively looking forward to it.

One of the last patients to have a check before Christmas was Chalky, the Westie with bronchitis. His cough was well under control now and, encouragingly, no one in the family had started smoking again. The only downside was that Chalky was not finding his half rations to his liking. He had taken to hanging around the dinner table at meal-times staring pleadingly at the family. I begged them to remain firm: he was already a lot thinner and looked years younger.

By Christmas Eve I had done as much as I could. There were a few owned animals still in hospital and they would have to stay because they needed intensive nursing. We had the usual broken pelvis and jaws in cats, and otherwise there were ten strays and a puppy, who was being spoiled rotten. The hospital looked lovely with lights and decorations everywhere and ribbons round the patients. At this time the whole place feels like a great big family and I love it!

It felt strange leaving the car-park and heading up the Seven Sisters Road, knowing that I was having Christmas off. Gabriel and the emergency nursing staff had got it all organized, though: they would sit down to lunch together after the in-patients had had theirs. I hoped it would be quiet for them and that there wouldn't be any sad accidents to spoil someone's Christmas.

The period immediately after the holiday is frequently frantic. No one likes to worry the vet, doctor or any other emergency service over Christmas Day and Boxing Day so they wait a few days. Immediately after Christmas and before New Year are 'hot points', when we may see patients coming through the door in numbers more akin to the height of summer. But not this year. It seemed that many people were taking ten days off and going away. We had the luxury of a nearly empty hospital and a few quiet days. I knew, from bitter experience, that this was also the lull before the storm of abandoned pets – unwanted presents. But that would be next week.

Gabriel had had a pleasant Christmas Day with the nurses and not been rushed off his feet. Boxing Day – traditionally busier – had also been quieter than usual. The problems we see after Christmas are similar I imagine to those facing GPs. Mostly to do with over-indulgence! Colicky pains, vomiting and diarrhoea, bones stuck in throats and so on. Four of us ploughed through the consulting with a succession of such cases. Although dogs and cats are capable of eating anything, their stomachs are not designed for the rich, varied diet to which we subject ourselves at this time of year. It's a recipe for disaster! In fact, one of the commonest causes of diarrhoea in animals is chopping and changing the diet too frequently. We might like to do this ourselves, but dogs are better off with a good-quality brand-name food that they like, and fed in the same amount daily. 'But he'll get bored with it!' people say. That's not often the case, though, and a healthy pet will enjoy the same food each day and not suffer from diarrhoea. This fact is demonstrated perfectly in the post-Christmas period when the results of not following good dietary advice flood in. It still seemed amazingly quiet though for the time of year and we couldn't blame the weather, which was unseasonably mild.

It seemed especially quiet since the TV cameras had gone. At the end of a long series we are always tired but when the cameras depart an atmosphere almost of mourning comes over the hospital and we miss the friends we have made.

As is so often the case, just as I am immersed in a gentle tide of routine cases something unusual pops up to dust the cobwebs off my brain. I was confronted with a West Highland White Terrier – not much more than a pup, at just over six months. He was owned by a retired couple, and had been a present from their son. While petting the dog Mrs Jamieson had noticed a hard swelling on his lower jaw. The next day I was feeling the same thing. Both lower jaws, but particularly the right side, were swollen and hard. I puzzled for an instant because I had seen this before – perhaps five or six years ago. I struggled to remember the name of the condition. I knew it was poorly understood and that there was no effective treatment. However, it tended to get better as the dog got older. I booked James in for an X-ray, telling the owners that this was the only way to be sure of what we were dealing with. There was also a slight possibility that it was a bone tumour.

Half-way through the next consultation the name of the Westie's condition leaped into my mind: cranio-mandibular osteopathy. And, like all fancy, complicated names, it hid science's basic ignorance as to what was going on. I knew I could count on the fingers of one hand the number of cases I had seen. When I got home I would get out the books and see what, if anything, had changed in the last few years. From what I seemed to remember, and especially as James was showing no symptoms of difficulty in eating, I was reasonably hopeful that, apart from having a swollen jaw, the little dog would come to no harm.

And all of a sudden the end of the year had crept up on us. As always, it had flown by. I could hardly believe it had gone so quickly. We had all had our share of triumphs and failures, of euphoria and heartache, but on balance I had thoroughly enjoyed myself.

On New Year's Eve, I took stock. More time with the family next year. I must get fit – I would join the local health club; being a vet needs stamina. And I would make sure I carried on learning as much as possible, something all of us would be doing. Could next year be even better? I certainly hoped so!

INDEX